Medical Advice and Life Book

YEOP AZMAN

(Muhammad Zeitsev bin Azman, MD BSc)

Title

Copyright

Dedication

Prologue

How to Get Proper Medical Treatment

Physical Health

I/O   2

Turmeric for (Almost) Every Type of Sick   12

Food of the Gods   16

I <3 Beans   19

Sage Wisdom   23

Ellagic is Berry Good for You   27

No Stress on Cres   29

How Antonia Took My Breath Away   36

Pain in Your Brain Making You Insane? TRAIN!   42

Anti-Aging: A Hot Button Issue   50

Mental Health

Everything is Binary | No Gray Areas in Life | Lifestyle of a Libra   55

Knowledge Yields Empathy   62

I Ergasia Fernei Vasana   66

Braining Too Quickly   74

Simple Habits to Make Yourself Smarter   80

In a Box   84

Social Health

Dulcius ex Asperis   **87**

Heal the World   **92**

Metabolic Placebo   **96**

"Loneliness is often the product of a gifted mind."   **105**

Environmental Health

Earth Day Star-date NOW!   **111**

This is The Rhythm of The Night...   **116**

Disclosure

Epilogue

About the Author

Published by Muhammad Zeitsev bin Azman, MD BSc

ISBN: 979-8841-0540-78

Cover design by Muhammad Zeitsev bin Azman, MD BSc

I would like to dedicate this book to **Danijel Dubičanac**, because he is the only one who read my writings, critiqued them to the point I got better at writing, was patient with my post-traumatic symptoms, edited and proof-read my mistakes *in English*, and was there to get me out of depression long enough to write.

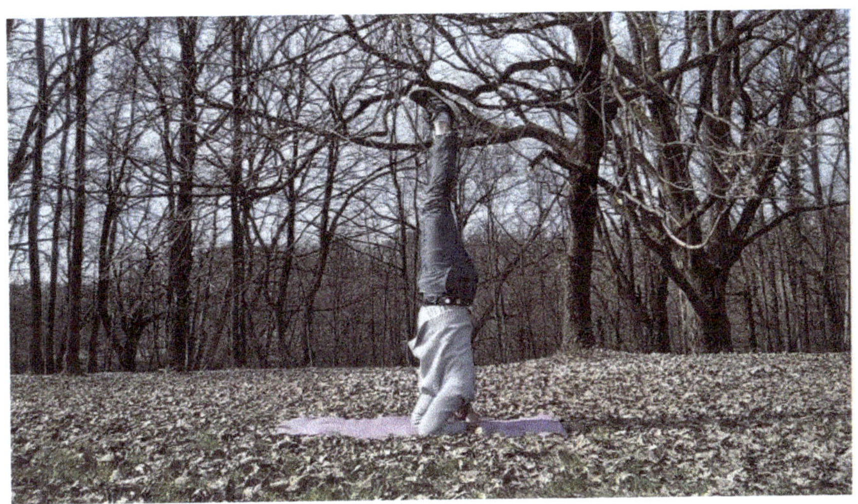

Prologue

In attempts to work on my writing and editing skills, I stared writing on my 31st birthday with alternative medicine as a subject matter. I researched to see what medical practices are good in the long run, and give advice on healthy living and preventive medicine.

In my recent applications to PhD programs in Public Health, I proposed to research the use of alternative life styles as preventive medicine to incorporate habits, that are considered alternative to conventional medicine, into every day behaviors.

It didn't work.

As most health-related lifestyle changes are hard to commit to, I believe that unhealthy vices can be balanced out with healthy ones. I am constantly aiming for **small changes** that will create the **biggest impact**. This will in turn promote a lifestyle of moderate usages and promote good health and longevity, a goal desired by most.

I will share this knowledge with you through short, easy-to-read essays explaining the benefits of aiming for a healthier lifestyle.

How to Get Proper Medical Treatment

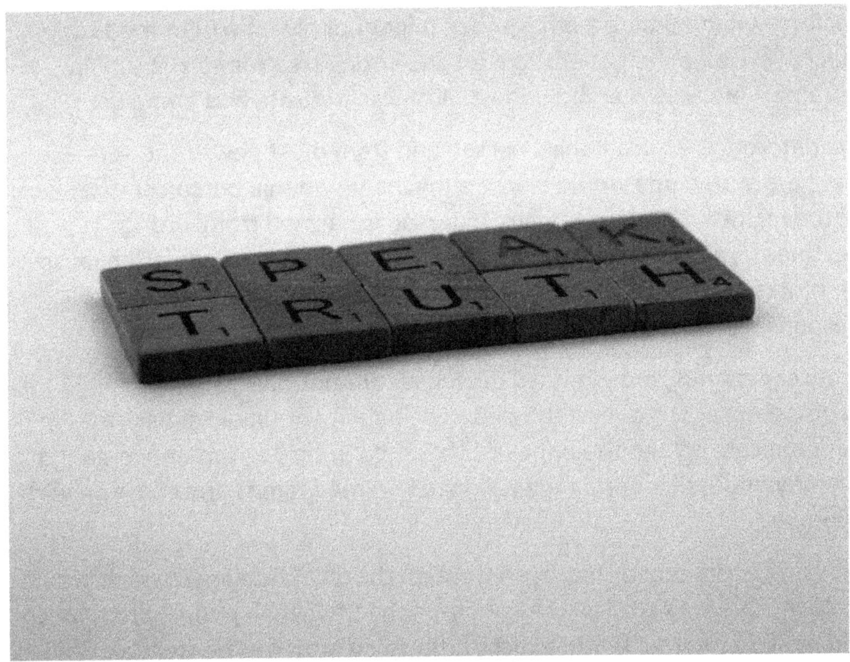

I read clickbait articles on MedScape about other doctors who get sued for either intentional or unintentional mistakes, and the lessons were always the same: Scare me into revising my thoughts multiple times before even making a peep to my patients.

Doctors have lost their respect with the general public, and I have seen mechanics get more respect when they mock their "patients" for abusing their cars. When we tell patients that they abuse their bodies, we would get complaints to our superiors, get financially punished, or even worse, fired for being honest.

I agree that there should be tact when dealing with that sensitive issue. After all, you should be sensitive about telling a 150 kg obese person that they should eat less. They might just sit on you.

People laugh when I compare doctors to mechanics, but there are very many similarities. They both fix the symptoms of the problems without fixing the cause. They both release people into the wild with the capability to harm themselves or others. They both are responsible for the source of the problem.

Mechanics, when they miss a screw, might not fix the brakes correctly, which will cause the car to swerve and crash; potentially harming a life. Doctors, when missing a differential, might not give the right medication, which will cause the patient to start the wrong treatment; potentially harming a life. Both can be honest. Both can educate and empower.

The difference – from a third person and from most news reporters – is that hardly anybody would blame a mechanic when a person crashes a car on the highway. However, when a person is harmed from wrong treatment, reporters, family members and the entire village will pick up pitchforks and torches to storm the hospital; ready to hang the one "responsible". Blood for blood.

In my experience, most missed diagnoses are not due to my incompetence, but due to the patients' inability or unwillingness to communicate. When the entire truth is hidden through shame or guilt, it is nearly impossible for a medical doctor to read minds and come up with solutions.

I am sure every doctor has been through the STD cheating chain. It would be so much easier to stop the spread of the STD when people are honest and bring in their ACTUAL sexual partners, so both can be treated. Guilt, embarrassment and cultural blocks are the mainstay of why doctors treat patients like statistics.

Mechanics do not have to know the entire story of why only the rear tires are bald. They just know it needs to be replaced, and they will replace it. In my experiences, most mechanics do not take the time to point-check other systems to make sure they need replacing. If and when these amazing mechanics do, they are also accused by their "patients" that they are mentioning fixes to increase the charges.

How many of us has had an alternator replaced, and have been advised to change the water pump at the same time? How many of us ignore that and let our engines heat up, so the mechanic has to take apart the same screws again? How many times did that water pump fail, drenched the alternator, and the mechanic had to tell you to replace the alternator that you JUST replaced a few hundred miles ago?

Do most patients listen to the advice of professionals before jumping to blame them for their own consequences?

Since people have stopped looking up at us as honorable advisors and healers, we have to heal with whatever information is presented to us. That leads to some unavoidable errors. Working in Emergency Medicine, I do not have the time to patiently wait for information. I also do not have the luxury of people bringing in their patient history and list of medications. I do not have access to hospital or primary health care data (at least in the form of ICD-10 (international code of diseases) list of diagnoses, current medications and allergies, so I just have to rely on the patients' inconsistent memories, and be ready with my anti-anaphylactic kit.

Thus, sometimes I rather empathize with my peers instead of reading about the "atrocities" of doctors' actions. We are paid too little to deal with lives of dishonest individuals. Fault should be given to the patient, as clues to illnesses are mostly based in patient history. That is why we were constantly barraged with learning clinical propaedeutics throughout our education.

Patients have to be 100% transparent. If they are not, they should not expect the correct treatment, because symptoms overlap.

In these cases, "I do not know." will not protect anybody.

Physical Health

I/O

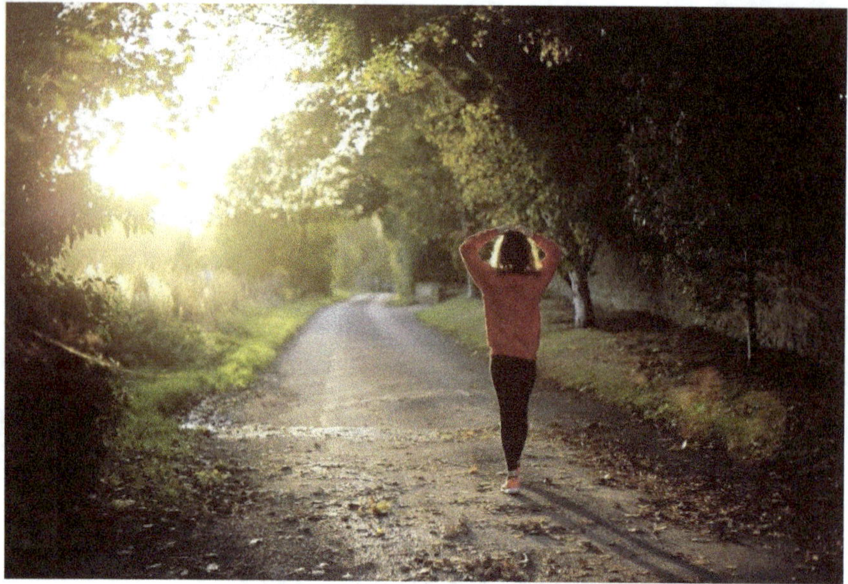

For most people, physical health is a hard goal to achieve. Health itself is a definition that not many people fully think about (until it is too late), as it involves separate components of physical, mental, social, environmental and sometimes spiritual health. Each component of health is highly intertwined, and to ignore one aspect of health would adversely affect the others.

There are many examples where mental, social, environmental and even spiritual health effects physical health. Without going into much detail and many examples; **leaded** products that disrupted mental development were banned, **CFCs** that destroyed the ozone leading to skin cancer caused by **UV** damages were banned, **asbestos** that directly caused lung cancer was banned, **deforestation** that dislocated animals that lead to more zoonotic jumps in diseases is being realized and reversed, realization and the fight against prejudice and **discrimination** allow more social groups to attain equality and equity, **mental changes** in mood that directly affect physical health are finally being less taboo, and much more.

People usually create goals of good physical health, and are barraged with advertisements of fad diets and fad exercise. Simplifying the concept of a healthy lifestyle into basic inputs and outputs can turn the currently confusing "goal" of good health into more of a "theme" of good health. Simplification is always a better option in terms of achieving a better quality of life. This ties overall concepts of health together in all aspects in this limited quantity of life.

Preventive medicine, in terms of physical health, is the balance of intrinsic factors (mainly genetics and culture) and extrinsic factors (mainly the inputs and outputs that balance the metabolism of the body). In the current industrial age, metabolic syndrome is the main issue plaguing modern medicine. Although today's society concentrates on harder medical problems, such as cancer and mental illnesses, metabolic syndrome is the root cause of the more common diseases that range from heart disease, stroke, diabetes, etc.

Metabolic syndrome is dependent on the body's genetic ability to metabolize the inputs (nutrients), and use those inputs for energy, to build and create other molecules, and to regulate excess. A lot of people, in this current sliver of human existence, live a life of excess. The body is then overwhelmed, and will store these excesses for future use. An earlier version of "us" can then have access to energy storage during harsher times.

Since there is no real need to uproot and migrate long distances on foot anymore, excess storage remains unused, and humans have eventually become nice marbled meat for stalking saber-toothed predators. On top of that, not regulating and balancing inputs and outputs can lead to a host of downstream issues, such as type 2 diabetes, circulatory problems and heart disease; the three common chronic "diseases" in today's society. These problems can compound further and evolve into neurological diseases, strokes and myocardial infarctions.

Although nutrition is not a simple topic (everything is always multi-factorial), there are many ways to prevent metabolic syndrome, balance input and output, and increase longevity and quality of life. There is a lot of advertising of dietary fads that do not cross cultures, exercise regimes that require massive changes to lifestyles, and a lot of monies spent on products that have ended up being expensive clothes racks.

However, there are simple habits that can be implemented in every lifestyle, which have been promoted by almost all Public Health sectors of every nation. Advertising, marketing and social media have unfortunately been louder than reliable sources, and so the illusion of choice is limited to the lizard brain of laypersons. Many do not question or research content, and blindly follow the shine and glamour of magazine covers displaying people who have probably access to personal trainers.

Most often, people spend billions of monies on products that can be replaced by knowledge and common sense. Cutting through the smokescreen of shine and glamour, these simple habits – which can be easily implemented into daily life – are ultimately distilled down to **eating well** and **exercising smart**.

Nutrition in a Nutshell

Nutrition is easy. Balanced nutrition is hard. As humans, we have been eating since we have evolved into modern humans. Some say that we have even started to eat before then. Probably an apple. That is probably why Adam and Eve did not need medical attention. Evolution, habits and migrations of our ancestors greatly affect the nutrients we require. In recent human history, globalization has influenced our bodies' biochemistries in efficiently metabolizing (or not metabolizing) certain foods.

Luckily, foods are not complicated. Macronutrients can be easily separated into fats, proteins, carbohydrates, alcohols, and healthy bacteria. Anything smaller are micronutrients. Even though the human body is evolved to biochemically turn molecules into fuel and structures, there are certain molecules and elements that even the complex human protein mechanics cannot create. These are the essential nutrients that are naturally found in different foods, which the body needs to grow and work well.

The body "burns" **fats** at 9 kCal/gram, **proteins** at 4 kCal/gram, and **carbohydrates** at 4 kCal/gram. **Alcohol** burns at 7 kCal/gram. According to UK's NHS and European Food Safety Authority (EFSA), men have to eat around 2400 kCal per day and women have to eat around 2000 kCal per day. The numbers are slightly higher in the USA. The calorie requirements depend on the age and growth of people, the intensity of activities and exercise, and some genetic factors that determine the rate of metabolism.

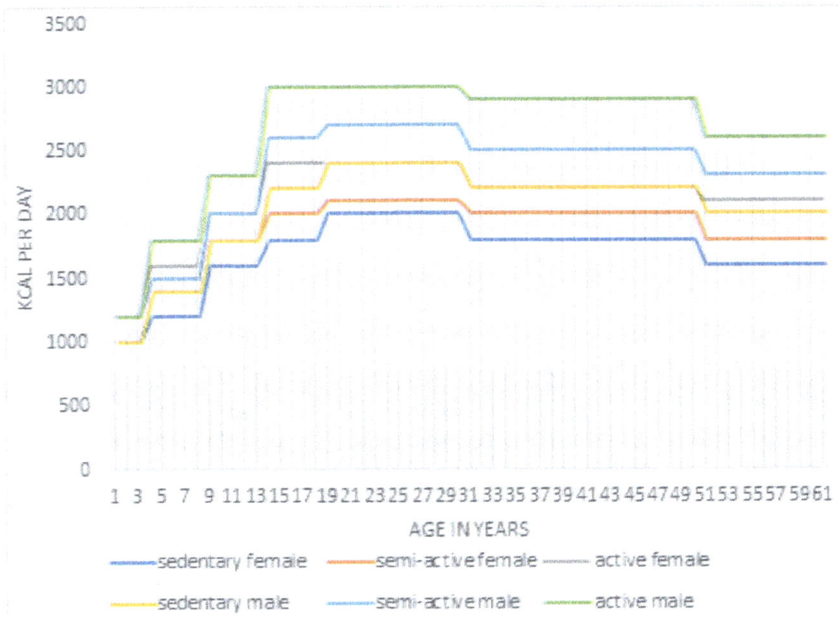

The basic ingredients to life could be balanced by fulfilling the caloric needs based on age and the body's requirements at that time. Interestingly enough, most cultures have foods that reflect the ratio of 1 fat : 2 protein : 2 carbohydrate. Taking the daily required calories and doing simple math with macronutrients, a medium McDonald's meal with orange juice is actually a calorie sufficient diet. Add in essential nutrients and fiber (a garden salad can be substituted instead of fries in some countries), and it can actually be a balanced diet.

McDonald's Medium Cheeseburger Value Meal		
Cheeseburger	119 g	313 kCal
Bun	57 g	150 kCal
Cheese	17 g	45 kCal
Patty	45 g	118 kCal
Fries	119 g	220 kCal
Potato	43 g	79 kCal
Oil	14 g	26 kCal
Orange Juice	460 g	190 kCal
Sugar	39 g	190 kCal

	Fat	Carbohydrate	Protein	Totals
Energy	9 kCal/g	4 kCal/g	4 kCal/g	
Ratio	1	2.25	2.25	
2200 kCal	400 kCal	900 kCal	900 kCal	
per meal	133 kCal	300 kCal	300 kCal	733 kCal
	15 g	75 g	75 g	
Meal	71 kCal	340 kCal	118 kCal	729 kCal
	31 g	139 g	45 g	

I didn't break down foods into the exact ratios of macronutrients. Fries throw the ratio of a meal to the fatty side. A garden salad can be substituted instead. Cutting out sugars by substituting the orange juice with water, coffee or tea (without much sugar) can also help balance the meal.

I chose a McDonald's meal to break apart, because it is standardized and contains separated ingredients. I am also currently eating it whilst writing this. Other meals can also be broken down into their respective macronutrients, but they all depend on preparation. That is why nutritional values of macro- and micronutrients is difficult to calculate.

The problem comes with the option of super-sizing, which is available at low costs. Our lizard brains will want to take the bigger (but not necessarily better) option, because humans are easily influenced by marketing. What people do not realize is that economists are paid millions to do market research to find the price that is worth losing for people, which can still be profitable for the companies. These prices are not randomly made, but researched to manipulate our minds into thinking we have a choice.

Remember that by falling for marketing, you are not saving $1.00. You are spending 50¢.

Although alcohols are never a necessary source of energy, fermentation of certain foods provides the body with some minerals, vitamins and antioxidants that are needed for a healthier lifestyle. Fermented foods are high in calcium, potassium, phosphorus, riboflavin, and vitamin B12. This is why most cultures have some sort of fermented foods, from kimchi to tempoyak to yogurt.

Fermented foods can also bring in good bacteria, such as Lactobacillus, through products like kefir, a fermented yogurt drink. Good bacteria are important to gut health. They are symbiotic to our body, and humans share this symbiosis by providing bacteria with things to eat. They then poop out nutrients for the gut to absorb. These bacteria also colonize the gut and create competition for space with bad bacteria, protecting your gut from infections.

Although hitting certain calorie goals is important for survival, people are starting to realize that instead of constantly metabolizing foods, an intermediate period of rest for the body allows metabolic processes (output) to keep up with the input. Intermittent fasting allows time for the cell to fix itself between metabolic events. As a person ages, pauses in input protects the cell by activating an enzyme called AMP-dependent protein kinase (AMPK). This protects the cell through downstream events involved in repairing, rebuilding, maintaining, and optimizing cellular structures and functions.

AMPK is involved in prolonging cell life by activating downstream enzymes responsible for cleaning the cell of reactive oxygen species, turning on genes that protect the cell from becoming cancer, giving time for the cell to fix errors in DNA, and killing damaged cellular components. Other enzymes are activated downstream, which increases glucose usage until there is no more glucose. That promotes fatty acid metabolism until there is no more fatty acid.

In antiquated cultures, being hefty is a sign of stability. In modern times, being hefty is just lack of common sense. With people dying from diabetic, cardiovascular, and neurological diseases, having a goal of being fat should not be associated with prosperity.

A friend once said that, "See this belly? Do you know how much money it took to get this?"

I replied, "See this six-pack? Do you know how much more time and money it takes to get rid of that belly?"

Being overweight not only exacerbates metabolic disorders, it gives the rise of symptoms and diseases that encompass metabolic syndrome. Although not a perfect way to monitor dietary goals, maintaining your body mass index (BMI) is much better than just measuring weight alone. As people have different cultures and have different goals, the main theme is to **eat healthier**. Considering current dietary habits, letting the stomach feel hunger and generally matching input with your output contributes to a more balanced and healthy physical life.

Exercise Made Easy

If you do not use it, you lose it. Aging is not a mental thing. 50 is not the new 30. Physical aging starts in your late 20s, and deterioration starts in your late 40s. As much as you try to control your cellular structure and metabolic processes with your mind (or soul or chakra or prayers), it won't happen. Without constant maintenance, muscles will begin to atrophy, posture will change due to laziness, things will start hurting out of nowhere, and the brain will forget where the keys are. We're ultimately biological machines that need regular checkups and oil changes. If we want to make our machinery last, we can always maintain functionality until it eventually shuts down.

As opposed to chronic diseases that adversely effects the body, maintenance of the body can lead to chronic health. Most symptoms of aging are reversible. The main symptom that leads us to lean forward and lose posture, stops us from doing medial tasks, and distracts us from exercising is pain. This pain comes from inflammation that react to signals released by aging and dying cells. The combination of the right nutrients, manipulating enzyme concentrations and the maintenance of physical structures of the cells making up the body is the key to happy longevity.

Exercise benefits the body by using the nutrients to replenish and rebuild old cells, and in the process allows us to burn and use our energy input. The human body goes through several activities during the day, each burning their own amount of calories. Even doing nothing burns calories, because cells like to live and they need energy to be born, grow, go to school, get a job, do the nasty and eventually die. Some cells even rebel (cancer) and that rebellion uses a lot more energy.

In order to do nothing – except breathing, beating your heart and maintaining homeostasis – a minimal amount of energy is used. This is called the basal metabolic rate (BMR). In general, the BMR can be calculated using the Harris-Benedict formula. The equation varies widely between genders, and taking average BMI between genders in the world, the mean calories burned is about 1600 kCal/day. Sleep burns about 50 kCal/hour, office work burns about 34 kCal/hour, and thinking uses about 320 kCal/day (although seeing how people are these days, I am surprised that they burn any calories at all). What's left is the energy that you have to burn to maintain weight.

Exercise more to lose weight. Exercise less to gain fat.

Follow the calories!

BMR – *1580 kCal/day*

Office work – *300 kCal/day*

10,000 steps – *around 350 kCal*

Total: *2230 kCal/day*

BMR is calculated by finding mean age (30), and calculating BMR from average mass (70ish kg) and average height (160 cm and 170 cm) for female and male. Thinking and sleeping are part of BMI and stagnant office work is "technically" rest, but I'll add it in. Total comes to the average input kCal, but most people would eat more or be REALLY sedentary. Some output is still needed for maintaining the physiology of your bio-machinery.

If the input is the recommended average of 2200 kCal, then a good hour-long walk is needed daily on top of working for monies. People can also compensate by eating less, but must take care not to skip out on essential micronutrients. Supplements can be used while calorie restricting, but reducing each balanced meal by 33% would be healthier. Intermittent fasting would be even better, because of its ability to "pause" metabolism, and allow the cell to fix itself.

If you cut out or burn an excess 500 kCal/day, you could effectively lose 1 lb per week. Losing up to 2 lbs (a little less than 1 kg) per week is safe, allows biochemistry to happen, and your mass won't easily bounce back.

As with any aspect of life, everything is multi-factorial. Nothing is that simple (it is). Nothing is binary (it is). Obviously exercising can be done to build muscle, but that has to be compensated by more protein-oriented calories. To be healthy and maintain muscle tone, good joint movement, a non-demented brain, and decrease that chronic pain that demotivates people from even getting out of bed, a simple routine of calorie usage (walking) and *anthropomorphic maintenance* (yoga) can greatly improve people's physical health. Done regularly, this can improve mental health. Done socially, exercise can also improve social and mental health.

Exercising is very easy.

People are just very lazy.

Public health sectors always advise daily activity. Being more specific, a 10,000-step regime throughout your day. In my personal experience, this is easily done working in Emergency Medicine. For me, ten thousand steps is about six miles. ***Note:*** *I am starting to like Imperial units for everyday measurements again.* This might seem like a lot, or people will always make the excuse that it does not fit in their schedule, but the point is to burn calories and to incorporate exercise into a lifestyle of stagnation.

Throughout the day – unless you have the lifestyle of bed to bathroom to car to garage to elevator to office to elevator to garage to car to couch to bed – you are bound to hit at least half of the daily requirement. This leaves just a few thousand more steps for a healthy daily routine anybody can accomplish with good company.

I am single :-(

Make it a habit, share the burden with someone you love, take it slow and build up, and eventually it gets easier. Mental stress will start melting away, and you'll feel better about yourself. If you can't find the time, make it shorter by jogging. If you are still making excuses, turn off your TV and go outside. Everybody seems to have more excuses than time.

A good supplement to walking is yoga. This is only a personal preference, but people can do Tai Chi or anything similar, or THOROUGHLY stretch after a warm up and before any longer activity. Yoga is old and hasn't faded, so it has merit. Yoga does not have to be linked to the rest of Ayurveda, but the series of movements concentrate on the biomechanics of the muscles and joints in your body. Physical manipulation of visceral areas also has been shown to improve breathing, circulation and digestion.

Danijel Dubičanac had a 30-day sun-salutation challenge, which I followed and learned the basic movements of sun-salutation. I realized that this helped with joint pain as I got older (plus the trauma of two car accidents that almost killed me). Since then, I have added basic yoga positions – plus breathing techniques – to tone and strengthen core muscles, stretch muscles and tendons, relieve stress on joints, and increase blood circulation.

Although there are various types of ways to burn calories, no matter what you are into, some general rules to remember when starting to exercise are: warm up before stretching, stay in your comfort zone, make your movements intentional, pick your legs up, use proper equipment to avoid injuries, lift with your legs, have a spotter, tuck and roll, follow through, one step forward and two steps back, keep your head up, keep your back straight, breathe...

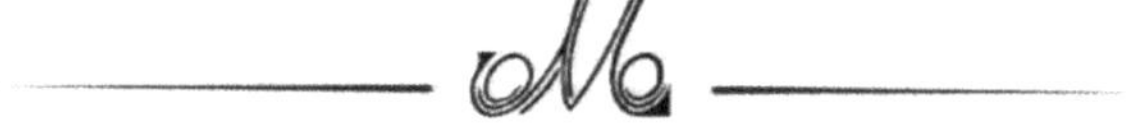

These concepts might be easy to understand; walk a hour daily with a friend or loved one, sincerely talk about your quality of life and learn something new with every conversation, eat a balanced diet and take care of gut health. That would cover physical, mental and social health.

Doing the calculations, I do not understand how people are overweight or even obese (unless there is an intrinsic reason). I struggle to eat 2200 kCal/day, and I have a habit of walking and biking instead of driving. It is so simple to stay within a normal range. I do not have gym muscles, but I have strength in the muscles that I use. Even when I was depressed, I was not sedentary enough to gain weight.

So how do people do it?

No judgement here.

Turmeric for (Almost) Every Type of Sick

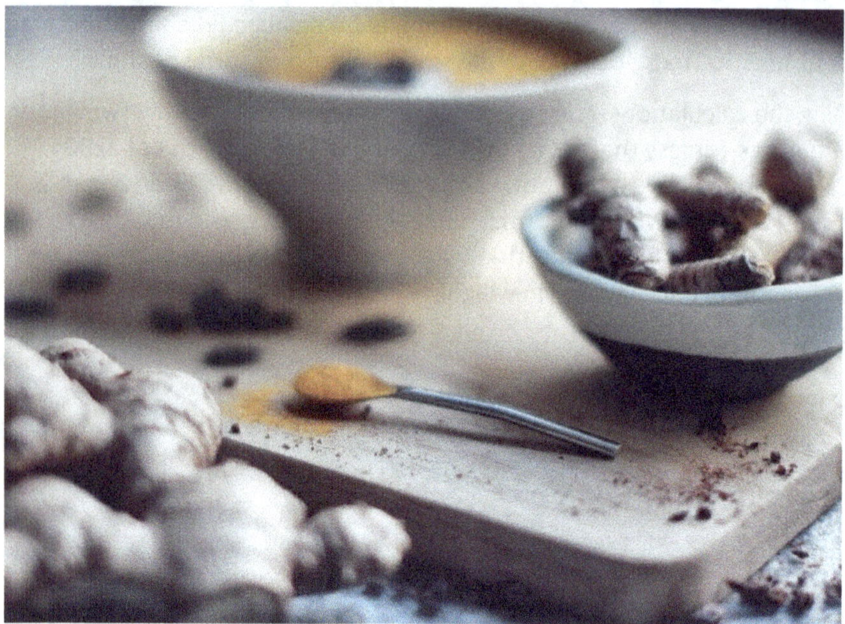

Alcohol consumption continues to become a constant issue, and abdominal pain seems to be a popular topic within the circle of people that seem to surround me. Within the realm of herbal remedies, there are a lot of natural products that help with regenerating liver function, helping with gastritis, alleviating pancreatitis and other alcohol-induced ailments.

Milk thistle seed extract and coffee enemas are two great remedies to treat an over-abused liver. However, I would like to introduce turmeric (*curcuma longa*) into the daily regimen of an alcohol connoisseur to counteract the long-term effects of alcohol.

Turmeric has been used in Ayurvedic medicine for over 3500 years as an antiseptic, an anti-inflammatory, an antioxidant, in skin ailments, etc. It has recently gained popularity within the past few years in conventional medicine as a potentially miraculous herbal remedy. This spice is native to the South Asian region and the majority of the world supply comes from Erode, a southeastern Indian city more commonly called the Yellow City.

As a spice, it is the main ingredient in curry powder and has been used for centuries in Asian cooking. The leaves of the turmeric root are also used in some cooking, although there is no mention of medical advantages from the leaf.

The main active substance found in the root of the turmeric plant is curcumin, the compound that gives the root its characteristic yellow color. Curcumin has been used for years as coloring for products ranging from cheese to soft drinks and is labeled E100 as a food additive. Although most of the research has been done in vitro and in animal studies, curcumin has been shown to have a variety of properties that is beneficial to medicine in human beings.

According to a few studies done within the past decade, curcumin is able to counter the effects of toxins through its antioxidant properties, inhibits the synthesis of inflammatory signals (eicosanoids), interferes with HIV P300/CBP binding sites, suppresses Herpes simplex virus-1 (HSV-1) replication by inhibiting RNA polymerase II recruitment to viral DNA, and also blocks HSV-2 in animal models of intravaginal infections. A study in 2004 has also shown that curcumin might also inhibit the accumulation of β-amyloid in Alzheimer's in animal studies.

A correlation study, measuring the mental state of elderly Asians who ate yellow curry, showed that their mini mental state examination (MMSE) scores were higher than those who ate less or no curry at all. In the study, there is no consideration of the other factors that contribute to good mental health. Curcumin also has a positive effect on the hippocampus and has protective properties against stress, depression and anxiety. More amazingly, this spice has been shown to be a selective MAO-A inhibitor, the same way some anti-depressants and anxiolytics work.

In addition to everything that has been previously stated, a study has shown curcumin to enhance the antibacterial effects of antibiotics against *S. aureus*. It also can induce apoptosis in cancer cells without affecting healthy cells. It has been shown that curcumin interferes with transcription factors, such as NF-kB, that can induce carcinogenic changes in cells. In a 2010 study done in Goethe University, curcumin inhibits malignant brain tumor proliferation, migration and invasion through interfering with the STAT3 signaling pathway.

Turmeric (*kurkuma*) powder can be found in most herbal stores and supermarkets. However, curcumin when eaten alone has little absorption and thus there is low bioavailability. Curcumin extract in capsule form increases the absorption of curcumin in the body by providing the compound in an oil-solubilized form.

This form is similar to most Indian curry preparations, and (for some people) would be a better alternative in complying with daily intake. Thus, I have included a recipe for a chicken dish originating from Erode that can be eaten with brown rice, a healthier alternative to common white rice. You can also try accompanying the dish with red yeast rice, which has a natural form of the cholesterol-lowering lowering drug, lovastatin.

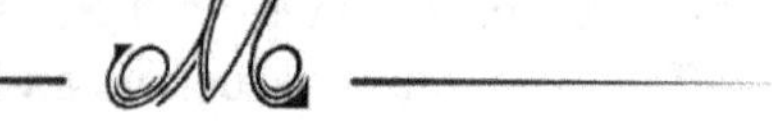

Pallipalayam Chicken Recipe

Ingredients:

1 kg chicken; I like dark meat, but if you use chicken breast, which is healthier, cut it into small, bite-size pieces.

2 large onions; finely chopped.

4 red chilies; seeds removed and broken into 3 or 4 pieces.

1 teaspoon of mustard seeds.

1 teaspoon turmeric powder.

1 or 2 curry leaves; bay leaves are a good replacement.

1 table spoon of chopped coriander leaves.

1 teaspoon of ginger and garlic.

2 tablespoons of oil.

Salt to taste.

Method:

Heat oil in a kadai or a wok and add mustard seeds. When the mustard seeds start to pop, put the chopped onions, red chilies and curry leaves. Sauté onions until they are slightly brown and then add the ginger and garlic and fry for a minute. Add the chicken, turmeric powder, salt and a sprinkle of water to moisten the mixture. Cover the kadai or wok and cook on a low flame until the chicken is fully cooked. Remove the lid and fry for about 5 minutes on low heat until you get a dry consistency.

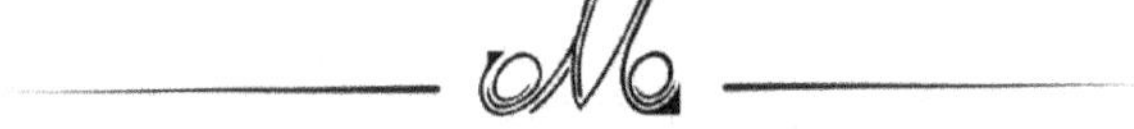

As I read more about turmeric in these newer studies, I stumbled upon a lot of possibilities for the spice and got excited by the research. Although eating curry every day is not a habit of mine, using a tablespoon of turmeric in daily cooking is not difficult to do. Since curcumin is available in a lot of food products already, it would be good to use these products on a daily basis.

Turmeric (like all toxin-eradicating antioxidants) is great at fighting the effects of alcohol, and a good, hot and spicy curry will help you with the morning after symptoms. As with all the other benefits of the spices found in curry, it is no wonder that the British soldiers carried the powdered form with them, allowing the masala or mixture of spices to travel around the world. Now you can find curry in every corner of the world, making this miracle spice (or mixture of spices) easily available!

Food of the Gods

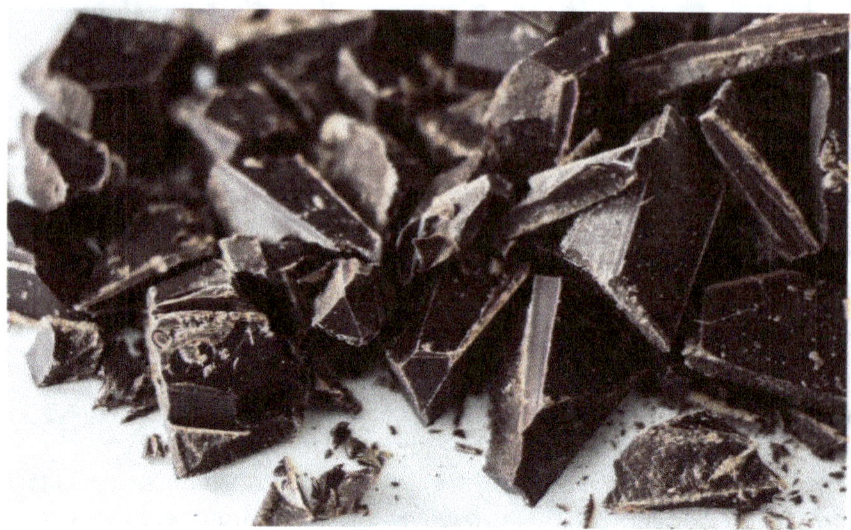

There has been a lot of research done on chocolate's effects on the cardiovascular system. I have to mention now that almost everything is good for something and most things are bad in excess. With that in mind, chocolate is a perfect example of a substance that needs to be taken in moderation. Why is chocolate good for your health? I can quickly answer that in a few paragraphs.

The reason why most of these "alternative products" are good for you is because of their antioxidant properties. Antioxidants are great at getting rid of toxins that cause oxidative stress on your system (which could lead to anything from atherosclerotic plaque formation to cancer). Being a powerful antioxidant, chocolate (as well as fruits, vegetables and teas duh!) has been linked to decrease chances of lung cancer by having a substance called plant-derived flavanol. Flavanol (not to be confused with flavOnol) lowers the risk of cardiac disease by increasing nitric oxide levels (NO), which lowers blood pressure.

Chocolate, or more specifically cocoa extract, is also linked to lowering ACE function in addition to increasing NO in your system. If you've ever had a heart attack, you would know that ACE inhibitors and NO sublingual pills are your best friends. ACE inhibitors and NO are used to lower blood pressure, a factor that is detrimental for the cardiovascular system. Since cocoa extract, the bitter part of BITTER chocolate (that some manufacturers remove to get rid of the bitter), mimics the effects of these drugs, it is easy to conclude the health benefits of chocolate.

However, chocolate has high amounts of low-density lipoproteins (the bad one). This is why eating normal milk chocolate is not very healthy for you. It's better to stick to the darker chocolate above 72%, which is available for an affordable price.

I, myself, love chocolate and if I start eating it, I can't stop. I would love to be a Kuna (not the Croatian animal or currency, but the people from Panama), because they drink cocoa from the early age of weening to death (at really old ages). As a reminder though, there are other methods in which you can lower your blood pressure.

I would suggest exercising regularly, quitting smoking, drinking a glass of wine, eating a square of chocolate, eating healthy ratios of macronutrients, buying yourself a bike and use it to get to work or college, and a lot of other great advice that most people do not comply to, which could get you to that level of health and quality of life.

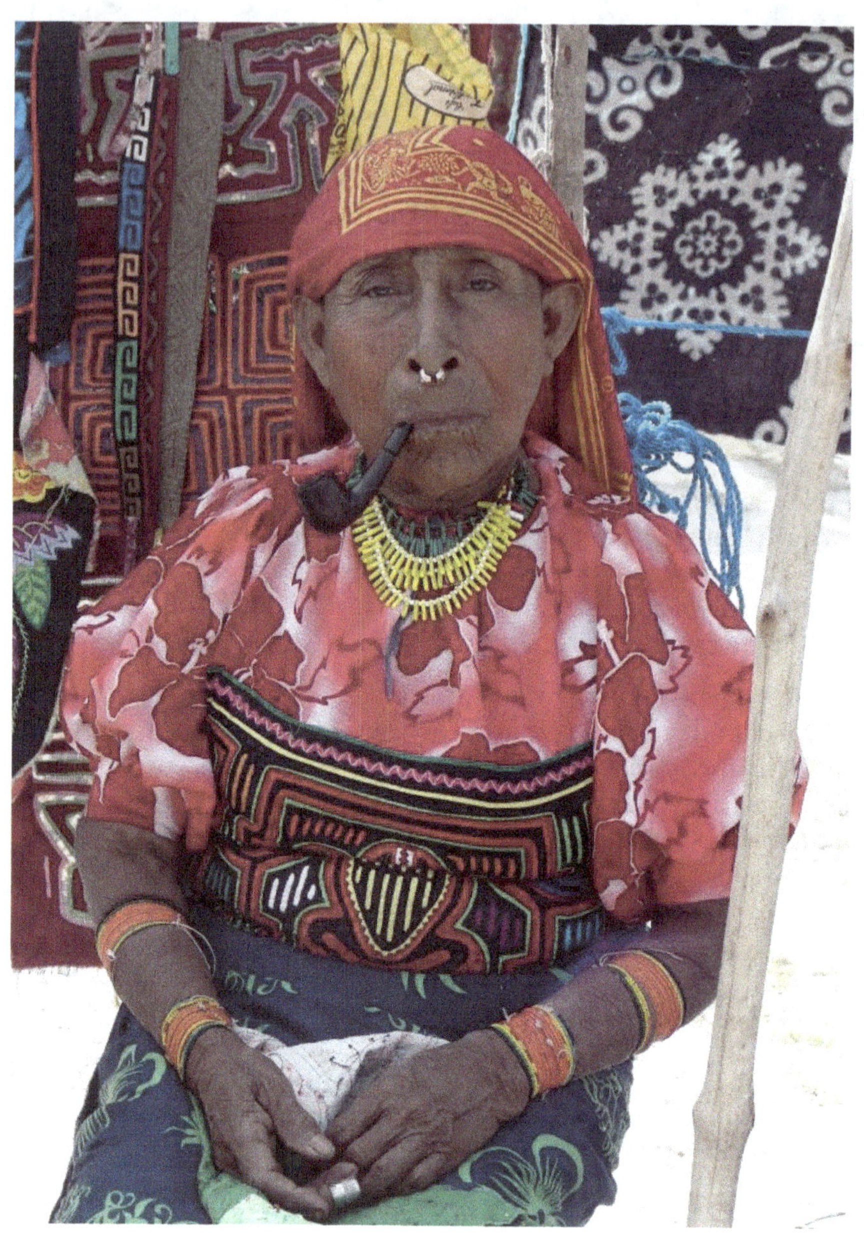

One kuna.

I <3 Beans

Being in Croatia for the past few years, and being a medical doctor has led to many questions. Some about infections; more about their genitals. The most questions I have gotten were about the health of their livers and their worries about alcohol consumption.

Most of the time and to keep questions to a minimum (after multiple annoyances), I simply reply with, "**stop drinking**." A lot of Croatians that I have met are considered alcoholics according to Western criteria by drinking more than 12 units a week; and going cold turkey is not really the best way to do it because of the consequences.

Although I do enjoy the occasional beer in this country, slowing down and drinking in moderation would be the best preventive step. However, most peoples' compliance to either abstinence or moderation is close to zero. I have found three solutions that alcohol consumers may or may not enjoy whilst trying to save their liver.

The **first** and most popular herbal remedy to recuperate the liver is milk thistle (*Silybum Marianum*) seeds. Milk thistle is native to the Mediterranean region and is in the family of daisies. The usage of the seed extract has been around for over 2000 years to treat cirrhosis of the liver.

This is mostly due to the silymarin content of the milk thistle seed extract. Silybin, the major constituent of silymarin, has protective effects on the liver and is used to repair damages ranging from hepatitis to alcohol to liver toxins such as *amanita phalloides* (death cap mushrooms).

Other functions of milk thistle include lowering cholesterol levels, reducing insulin resistance in people with type II diabetes who also have cirrhosis, reducing the growth of cancer cells in breast, cervical and prostate cancers, reducing the effects of a hangover, and reducing liver-damaging effects of chemotherapeutic drugs.

Since it takes about 7 kilograms of milk thistle seeds to make 1 kilogram of extract (maximum daily dosage is 800 mg), and that this is mostly **preventive medicine** and has to be taken daily, I would suggest getting silymarin capsules. Each capsule contains 150 mg and the recommended daily dose is 280 mg.

The **second** herbal remedy that is used to treat liver dysfunction is the Siberian ginseng (*Eleutherococcus senticosus*), a plant native to the Northeastern Asian region. Although the Siberian ginseng, more commonly called eleuthro, is very different from traditional Chinese ginseng in composition and structure, it is still an adaptogen (a substance that increases the body's response to stress) that has very similar effects to ginseng. Eleuthro thus increases endurance, improves memory function, has an anti-inflammatory effect, and is immunogenic. It is also somewhat chemo-protective and radio-protective; probably due to its immunogenic effects.

According to some articles, eleuthro is also much more effective than Chinese ginseng for its antioxidant properties. This is helpful in reducing the levels of toxins, such as alcohol, from the body. Eleuthro also has a few polysaccharides that enhance liver function and reduces the levels of certain enzymes that inhibit proper liver function. Since this ginseng substitute is better at ginseng functions than traditional ginseng, naturally it is difficult to find in Croatia.

The **third** and more directed to a perverted sense of herbal remedy is the coffee enema. An old "alternative" medical technique, coffee is used to detoxify the liver by draining the toxins from the entero-hepatic circulation. The coffee causes the toxins to remain in the colon instead of getting reabsorbed to be processed in the liver.

The caffeine also causes the bile duct to empty into the digestive system, thus allowing more toxins from the gall bladder or liver to be expelled. By removing toxins through the coffee enema, the liver has more capacity to handle the toxins in the body. Theoretically, reabsorption from the colon is disrupted. There *might* be a possible positive effect on reducing the amount of fats and cholesterol in the system, and also potentially increasing bile function.

According to *s.a. Wilson's Gold Roast Coffee*, who states that they are the best coffee for enemas due to their high caffeine and palmitic acid content, enemas can be done as often as possible to eradicate the effects of the toxin. Their recommended directions are:

Empty 4 cups of filtered or distilled water into a non-aluminum pot or saucepan. Add 3 rounded tablespoons of organic coffee (finely ground and not instant), preferably s.a. Wilson's Gold Roast Coffee. Stir the coffee to make sure all is mixed in the water, and then bring to a boil. Boil the coffee for 3 to 5 minutes whilst stirring occasionally. Reduce heat and cover pot or saucepan with lid and let it simmer for 15 to 20 minutes. Remove the pot from the stove element and let coffee cool down to room temperature or cooler. Strain the coffee through a fine sieve to remove as much of the coffee grinds as possible. Avoid using a paper or cloth filter to strain your coffee as it removes much more than the grounds, much of the prime elements, such as cafestol, will be lost by using cloth or paper. Because of the boiling process, some of the water may have evaporated. Add plain filtered or distilled water to the coffee to bring it up to 4 full cups.

Clamp the end of the enema bag and pour 1 cup of the filtered coffee mixture into the enema bag. Release the clamp until the coffee begins to flow out, and then clamp the bag again immediately. Hang the enema bag at a height of a meter. Lie on the floor and gently insert the nozzle, using vegetable oil on the nozzle if needed. Release the clamp and let the coffee mixture flow into the sigmoid colon. Clamp the tubing as soon as there is a sensation of "fullness" or when the enema bag is empty. Remove the nozzle. If possible and without forcing yourself, retain the enema for 10 minutes, and then empty your bowel. After emptying your bowel, repeat the process with the remaining cup of coffee. If you cannot hold one cup of coffee mixture enema, take several smaller enemas.

When the bile duct empties, you will feel a squirting sensation in the area of your right rib cage. After feeling the bile emptying, you can stop taking enemas for that day. If you do not feel the bile duct emptying after one week of daily enemas, increase the strength of the coffee or take slightly larger volume enemas. You should not feel nervous or jittery after the enema because the coffee does not get absorbed systemically. If you feel nervous or jittery, have palpitations or irregular heartbeats; reduce the amount of coffee by half or more. Repeat enemas as needed.

To explain things further, cafestol is a potential anticarcinogen that has shown to inhibit the progress of Parkinson's disease and also blocks cholesterol homeostasis and increases serum cholesterol by 8%. I am unsure how effective cafestol is when taken through the pooper.

Palmitic acid is a fatty acid that is also used in napalm and paliperidone. If taken with a good diet high in HDL, palmitic acid has no hypercholesterolemic effect. However, with an unhealthy diet, palmitic acid increases LDL, decreases HDL and has a harmful effect to the cardiovascular system.

This is why s.a. Wilson's Gold Roast Coffee has a motto of being "recommended by more professionals than any other single brand of coffee". Funnily, they did not specify the purpose or mentioned the quality of their roast in terms of great taste or aroma like the other coffee companies do.

In short, when you have a hangover after a night of going out and feel like alcohol has won another fight against your liver, take a few milk thistle seed pills, brew yourself a *cup of Joe* and get ready to spend the morning on the toilet. Which doesn't seem like too much of a lifestyle change.

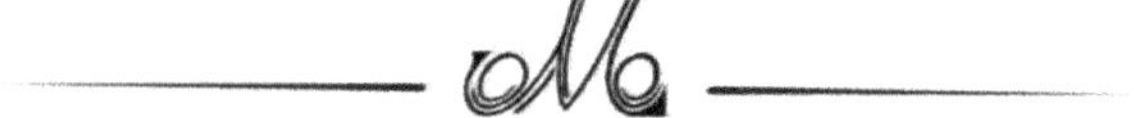

*I do **NOT** recommend a coffee enema. This is for information purposes only.*

Sage Wisdom

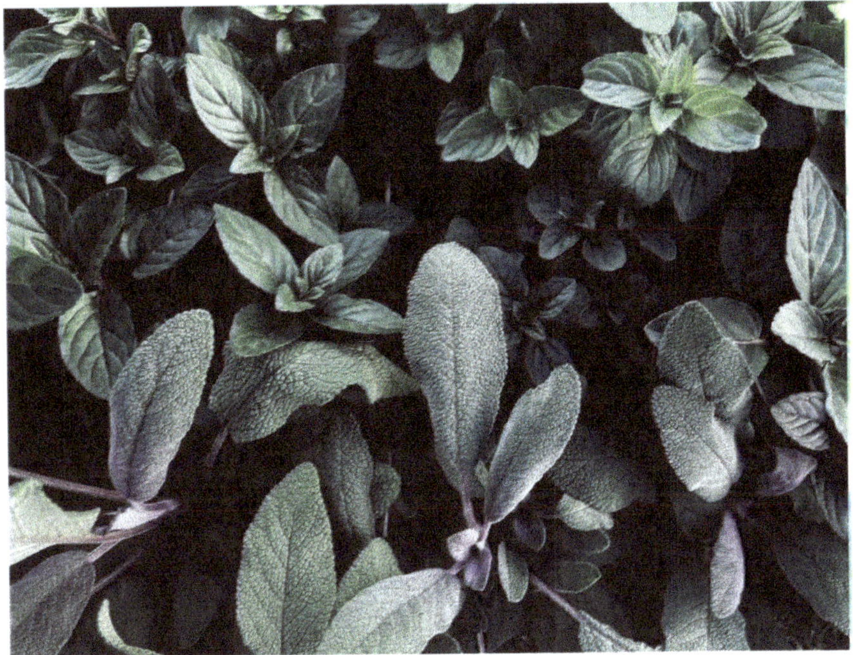

Salvia officinalis.

In the kitchen, sage has a slight peppery flavor, possibly due to the camphor flavor of eucalyptol, one of the major constituents in sage. Sage is great for flavoring fatty meats, poultry or pork stuffing, sausages, and in sauces. It is very popular in Adriatic and Mediterranean cuisines. Common sage is grown in many parts of Europe for the distillation of its essential oil.

Most of the time, herbal medicine is linked to Asian, South American or African cultures. However, sage is a native Mediterranean herb, and has been used for millennia by Romans for warding off evil, treating snakebites, increasing women's fertility, etc. Recently, sage was found to be effective in the management of mild to moderate Alzheimer's disease by inhibiting acetylcholinesterase, an enzyme that breaks down acetylcholine. This potentially increases neurotransmission and reduces the effects of dementia.

The constituents that are the most active in sage are eucalyptol, borneol and thujone. The sage leaf contains tannic acid, oleic acid, ursonic acid, ursolic acid, cornsole, cornsolic acid, fumaric acid, chlorogenic acid, caffeic acid, niacin, nicotinamide, flavones, flavonoid glycosides and estrogenic substances.

As a Local Antiseptic

As far as I have read, the most useful usage of sage would be as a local antiseptic. The main constituents that are the most active in sage are eucalyptol, borneol and thujone. These three compounds have great natural antiseptic properties. However, as with most natural products, there are many other compounds that are unaccounted for and could cause harm in excess usage.

The first compound that is good for antiseptic properties is **eucalyptol**. Eucalyptol comes from the essential oil of eucalyptus, but is also found in many aromatic herbs such as camphor, laurel, bay leaves, tea tree, mugwort, sweet basil, wormwood, rosemary, sage, and other aromatic plant foliage. It is a main ingredient in most mouthwashes, and is also used to control mucus hyper-secretion and asthma through inhibiting inflammatory reactions. Because of its good anti-inflammatory effect, it is also good in controlling sinusitis, reducing headaches and reducing nasal obstruction.

Borneol is used in moxibustion, an eastern alternative technique, in which the person's acupuncture points are heated to create natural blood and qi flow. Although I can understand physiologically how blood flow increases to the area of the skin when heated, I do not understand the concept of a flow of spiritual energy.

Let's explain why borneol is good for antiseptic properties using my knowledge of biochemistry and medicine. By increasing the blood flow to the area by vasodilation, borneol promotes the body's natural immune response. Borneol is also a natural insect repellant, but is found in higher concentrations in *Artemisia* (wormwood), *Blumea balsamifera* (sambong), and *Kaempferia galangal* (kencur). Not surprisingly, these plants are used as natural insect repellants, natural diuretics, and they are good for increasing immune response against the common flu and cold.

The third compound, **thujone**, is also used in herbal medicine to stimulate the immune system. Thujone affects the central nervous system, and the reported side-effects from the essential oil include sleepiness and anxiety. Thus, caution is indicated when using sage in conjunction with central nervous system stimulants or depressants.

Since thujone's chemical structure is similar to cannabis, it was labeled in the 1970s as a cannabinoid. However, it has been proven not to activate the same receptors that THC activates, but has been found to act on GABA and 5HT3 (nicotinic acetylcholine) receptors, which are responsible for inhibitory reactions in the brain and also excitatory pathways that cause anxiety.

Thujone, however, is famous for being an active compound in absinthe, although absinthe is made with another source of thujone, *Artemisia* (wormwood). Absinthe that is produced under the European Union have limits of maximum of 10 mg of thujone/L if there is more than 25% alcohol, and 35 mg of thujone/L for bitters with less alcohol. Knowing the historical effects of absinthe and alcohol, needless to say, thujone is reported to be toxic to both brain and liver cells, and could cause convulsions if used in too high a dose.

Maximum thujone levels for other products in the EU are:

0.5 mg/kg in food not prepared with sage and non-alcoholic beverages.

5 mg/kg in alcoholic beverages with 25% alcohol.

10 mg/kg in alcoholic beverages with more than 25% alcohol.

25 mg/kg in food prepared with sage.

35 mg/kg in alcohol labeled as bitters.

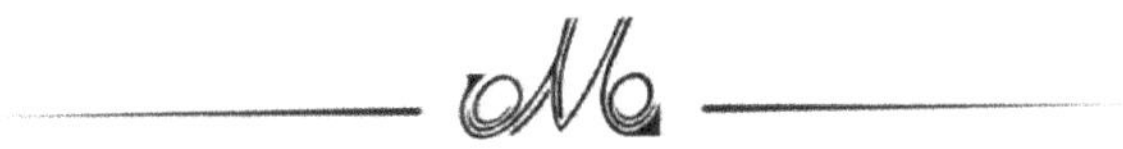

Knowing this, the three main compounds found in sage are great for fighting infections in localized areas. This is why sage is one of the main ingredients in a recipe called **Four Thieves Vinegar**, which I recommend to have in every household. Historically (legend), the Four Thieves Vinegar was used in France by thieves that would rob people who have the plague. The story states that they were caught, but did not have the plague despite being regularly exposed. In return for their freedom, they agreed to share the recipe of their immune system boosting concoction.

To prepare the Four Thieves Vinegar, use equal parts thyme, rosemary, sage, and lavender. Place herbs in a jar and cover with vinegar. Seal the jar and place it in a cool, dark place for six weeks. Strain the mixture into a spray bottle or a clean jar and use it as a disinfectant. All the ingredients have strong antibacterial agents. Add garlic for added strength, or if you're Chinese or Italian.

For Your Teeth

To answer a question on why gargling sage is good for your teeth; eucalyptol is used in mouthwash products, and is also a natural antibacterial. Borneol will also bring a good immune response. Thujone also has been proven to kill cells in vitro. The mixture of all three constituents would be great in creating a homemade mouthwash. You can also whiten your teeth with sage and salt, where sage and salt act as a natural scrubber. That doesn't mean that you can't create the same mouthwash using wormwood, eucalyptus or rosemary, etc.

To create the sage toothpaste, use a mortar and pestle to grind a handful of sage and a handful of sea salt together. Then bake the whole mixture in the oven (on a baking sheet or in a ceramic oven-safe dish). The shape of the mass does not matter; just bake it until it hardens. Grate the hardened mass of sage and salt until it turns into a powder. Store the powder in a short, wide-mouthed (preferably resealable) jar near your bathroom sink and use this powder instead of toothpaste.

However, I would still recommend brushing your teeth with toothpaste, because of the lack of fluoride in the sage-salt mixture. I was also trying to think of a clever name for the toothpaste, but couldn't think of anything.

Ellagic is Berry Good for You

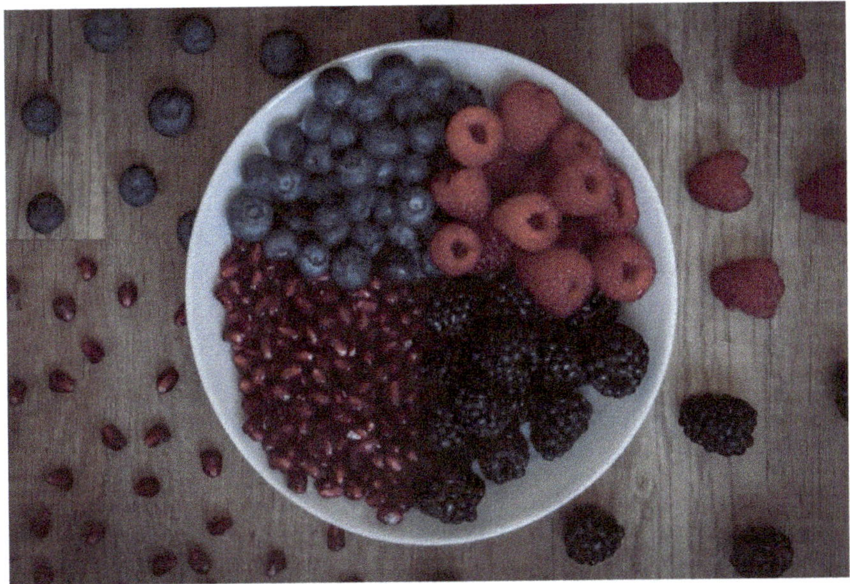

Being a smoker who is constantly on the verge of quitting, I came across an interesting article in one of the many publications that I read that states that strawberries have a substance called "ellagic acid" which activates p53/p21 expression that leads to a stop in cell cycle and causing apoptosis.

What does that mean?

That means, like anything else that has the potential of stopping cell replication and causing apoptosis, ellagic acid is "great" for preventing cancers, especially of the lung, colon, prostate, esophageal, and liver cancers; although the research is limited. In one paper, it states that you have to gavage strawberries to the point where you have to use the word "gavage" to describe how many strawberries you have to eat for it to be effective.

Ellagic acid is also in most other berries and walnuts, and after more research has been done on rats, and human trials will start (still new on the scene), there will always be people making supplements to get an easy buck until the FDA shuts them down for doing something stupid without putting proper research in their place.

Back to the point of promoting berries, nuts, and eating like a chipmunk, I realized that I haven't really explained what ellagic acid is. Ellagic acid is a phenolic compound that is derived from ellagitannins, which is conjugated in the stomach and absorbed as ellagic acid.

Why is that important? It's not unless you are doing research. The most important thing to know is that it helps in reducing the rates of cancers. It is also a potent antioxidant (like most natural foods the world), anti-inflammatory, and "wonder" substance.

One goal is to restore the health of the cells lining your lungs. All *antioxidants* will help, especially if combined. The most potent are curcumin, hesperidin, quercetin, ellagic acid, catechins, ferulic acid, anthocyanidins, and luteolins. These are found in grape seed extract, white tea, celery, kale, brussels sprouts, broccoli, oranges, and grapefruits.

I will constantly repeat that **preventive medicine is the best medicine**, and if you eat a balanced diet of vegetables, fruits, berries, nuts, curry, olive oil and other generally healthy foods, you can be sure that there will be something going on in your body that will help you out.

In addition to nutrition, I say that physics go a long way; expanding your lungs by breathing exercises and increasing circulation within your blood vessels give a chance for these wonderful antioxidants to work.

No Stress on Cres

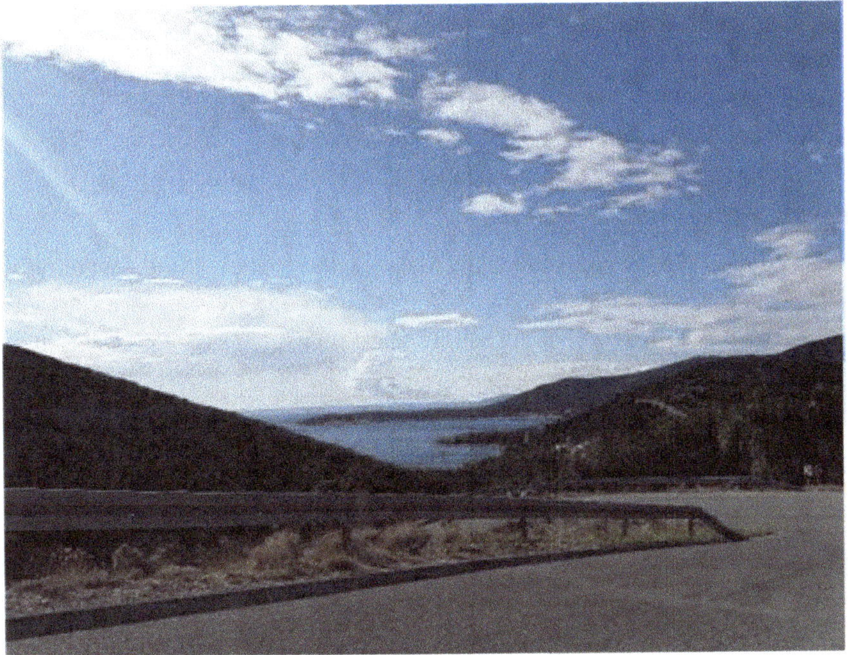

Heart-shaped bay of Martinščica

I moved to Cres the weekend before the 1st of July. I was in the City of Cres and waited for my colleague to come and drop me off in Martinščica, a small outskirt camping town and docking marina on the west coast of the Island of Cres. As we pulled into the tiny town with a little over 100 local inhabitants, I immediately fell in love with the heart-shaped bay and the collection of houses that line the coastline after the serpentine drop from main road on the top of the hill (9 km of windy roads to the coastline).

I immediately felt relaxed and let my guard down as we sat at Sidro (a café) with a hyperactive nurse from Rijeka. After a few dips in the sea, my colleague left and left me alone to open the small tourist clinic in the middle of Martinščica. My nurse, full of energy, decided to clean up nature and made me pick up all the pine cones, basically to make the clinic more presentable. However, she quickly lost will and energy, leaving me to finish cleaning up the exterior and to clean up the trash that was littered by the people who trimmed our trees.

I also lost a lot of energy and soon began to take more and more naps outside. The temperature got warmer and the only way I could snap out of it was to jump into the sea, which was at that time a crisp 20 degrees (Celsius). Bura, a cold westward wind coming from the mountains, was blowing cooling down the temperatures, but still I felt like something was always dragging me down. I slowed down on smoking, which usually gives me a bunch of energy. Nothing was working and I became worried.

Then on one EARLY morning (thanks to mosquitoes), I woke up to a wonderful smell that filled the clinic and decided to go jogging, since the morning was cooled down by a drizzle from the night before. I suddenly realized that it was a mixture of different aromas and narrowed it down to the aromas of pine, rosemary, lavender and immortelle.

My sister, who is into aromatherapy, got me curious about alternative, hippie techniques and therapies to sometimes disprove her methods, but more importantly find a reason why they seem to work. I have always used lavender as a sleep aid, and during that morning jog, I realized that this entire island is full of wild lavender, rosemary, immortelle and pine. That did not help my energy level as I took deep breaths of aromatherapy during my 3-mile run. I eventually came back to the clinic, showered and passed out until my first patient woke me up from my aromatherapy-induced nap.

I also learned from a newly-acquainted friend, who is from Martinščica, that there were cases of people with asthma or chronic obstructive pulmonary diseases that have left Cres cured of their symptoms.

According to Cres-Adventure.com (a website that no longer exists), Cres has the least inhabitants per square kilometer in the whole of the Mediterranean. Therefore, there are a lot of preserved flora and fauna. Since it falls on the 45th parallel, Cres has both continental and Mediterranean climates, so the island flora ranges from evergreens to pines to seasonal plants.

Pinoideae

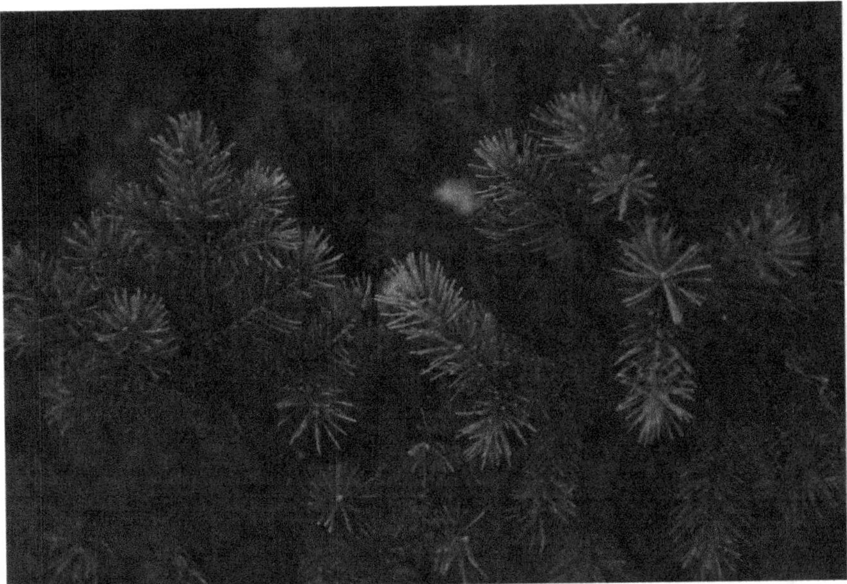

Pine is good for bronchial infections as it is both antibacterial and an antiseptic. Making an oil out of pine for aroma therapy can fight against lower respiratory infections. Pine oil also works as an expectorant, breaking up mucus and clearing it out from your lungs.

Steam inhalations work the best to clear up the lungs, but because the Island of Cres is covered with pine and the aroma is carried through salty winds, the people living on this island are constantly breathing in aromas of pine and its beneficial properties. Pine is also a great muscle relaxant, which is probably why I am having trouble getting motivated to move about and jog or bike.

Helichrysum italicum

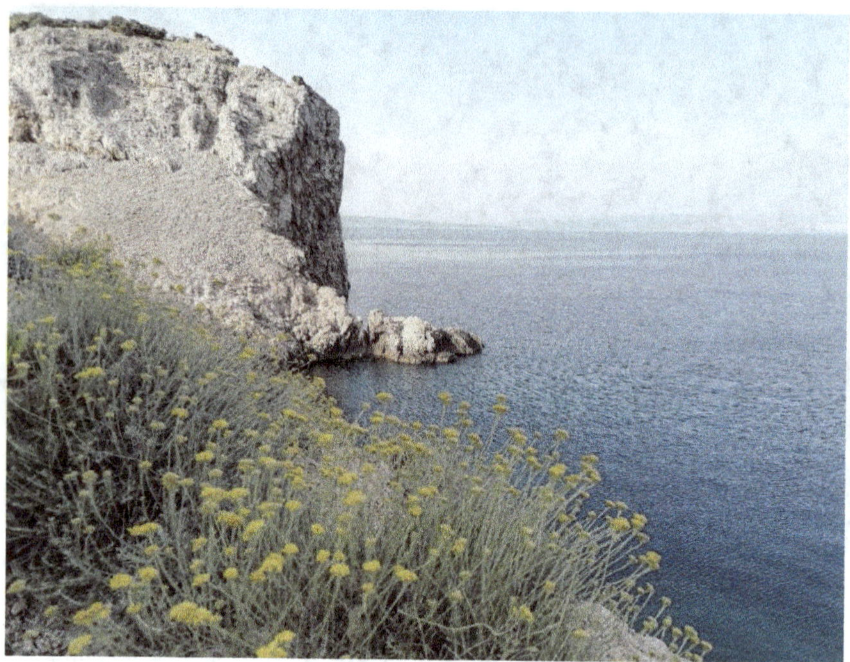

When my colleague, who had a summer house on Cres, said that she missed the smell of Cres, I didn't get it at first. Then she went to explain the smell of this yellow flower and looking into it, I found out that she was talking about immortelle. I didn't even realize these flowers were EVERYWHERE, but after going two steps into the nature, I found FIELDS of them. Immortelle gets its name from staying the same shape when they are dead and dried.

Oils made from this flower are rich in italidone, a ketone that helps in the absorption of hematomas and has an effect on tissue regeneration. Traditionally, immortelle is used for asthma, liver problems, migraines, psoriasis, dilated veins, etc. As an inhalant, immortelle can also break apart mucus, reduce irritating coughs as well as having an inflammatory effect.

According to Dr. Nina Bašić-Marković, the peppery smell of immortelle also invigorates the mind and reduces lethargy and depression. Since the clinic is surrounded by a field of immortelle, I am very unsure about that as we lose a lot of willingness to work.

Lavandula

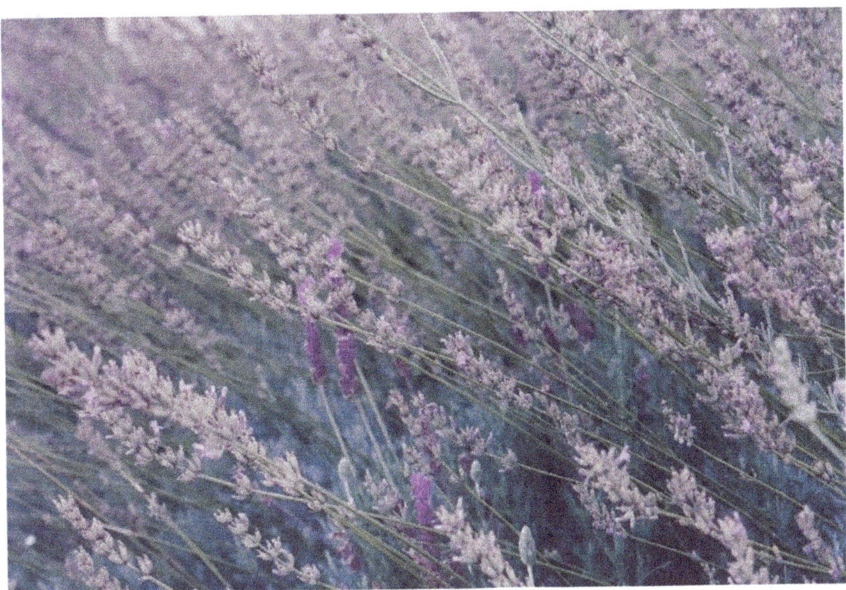

Lavender can be found all over the Mediterranean and is known for its anti-mosquito properties (although it never works), its sleep-inducing properties and its amazing ability to keep moths away from clothing. Due to high levels of camphor and esters, essential oils are not suitable to be used with small children and pregnant women. One article mentions that lavender is great for the common cold, rhinitis, cough and sinusitis.

Its aromatic properties have the same effect as pine and immortelle, adding to the muscle soothing and pulmonary healing effects. However, lavender has a sedative effect on the heart muscle, and thus is great for high blood pressure, palpitations and tachycardia. Being an antiseptic and analgesic, lavender is an ideal choice for treating burns and reducing scarring. Besides many other uses, the most important effect of lavender is its ability to reestablish balance to the mind and the body.

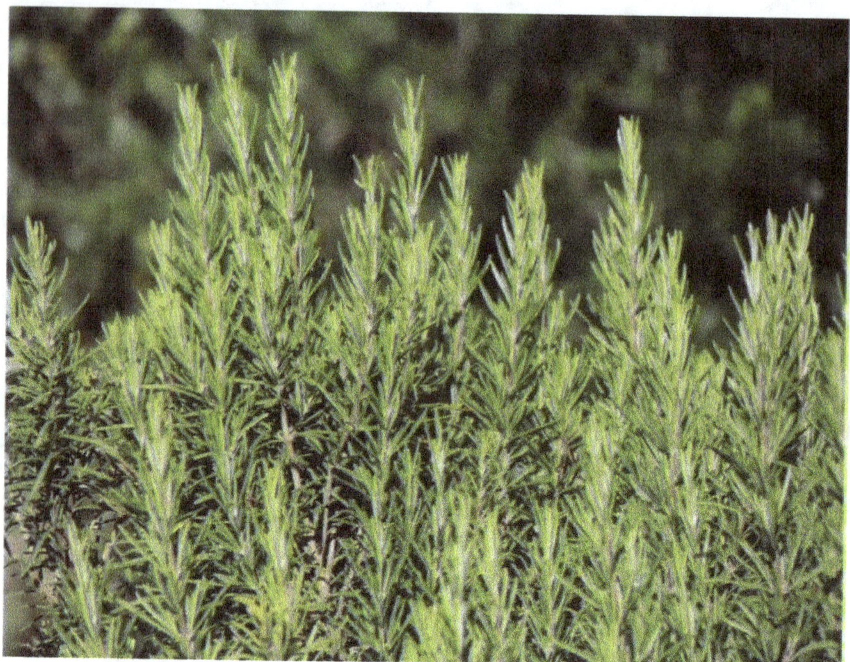

It is believed that rosemary strengthened memory, and is also the symbol of fidelity. The smoke from burnt rosemary was inhaled to protect against brain weakness and dizziness, and the herb was burned in schools and universities to inspire the pupils. Until the twentieth century, the branches were burned with juniper in French hospitals to purify the air. Rosemary is abundant in the Mediterranean and blooms in late winter and can be found very close to the sea.

Rosemary, like many other natural plants, is full of esters and aromatic - *ols* that serve as an antiseptic, astringent and antioxidant. This plant can relieve rheumatic and muscle pain, relaxes nerves, improves digestion and appetite, and increases sweating. Vapors from its essential oil can reduce congestion and stimulate the nervous system to increase energy. It can encourage old, dry skin to produce its own natural oils and reduces canker sores.

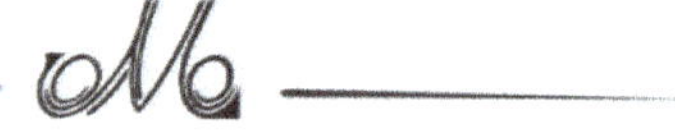

I realized that the aromatic mixture of these four plants have increased my lung capacity, and I do not feel the need to smoke. I can breathe better, but my muscles are so relaxed that I do not feel like jump-starting anything. With this in mind, I think I found the perfect mix to have whenever you have a hard day at the office, or if you have sore back and a significant other to rub oils onto your back.

I have neither.

I decided to make my own Cres mixture of aroma therapy, and see if I can recreate this relaxing sensation for my friends. Looking up on Wiki How, I found a simple way to create a mixture of these four herbs and see if there is something to this alternative medicine aromatherapy doo-hickey!

Sterilize your jars and lids

Place them in a large pot of boiling water for around 5 minutes

Allow the jars and lids to cool and air dry.

Choose your herbs

Chop up enough of the fresh herbs to fill up the jar.

Fill the jar with the freshly chopped herbs, and compress them.

Heat about 0.250 L of light unscented oil in a small saucepan until it reaches 71.1°C.

Use a meat or candy thermometer to obtain a precise reading.

Pour the hot oil over the fresh herbs in the jar.

Use the knife blade to move the oil and herbs around to release any air bubbles and to seal the lid.

Allow the jar to cool until you can handle it.

Use a label and marker to indicate what blend is in the jar.

Pick a cool, dark place to store the jar for at least 1 month.

The oils from the herbs will infuse with the oil in the jar to make essential oils.

Aromatherapy essential oils must be stored in the dark to prevent light from breaking them down.

How Antonia Took My Breath Away

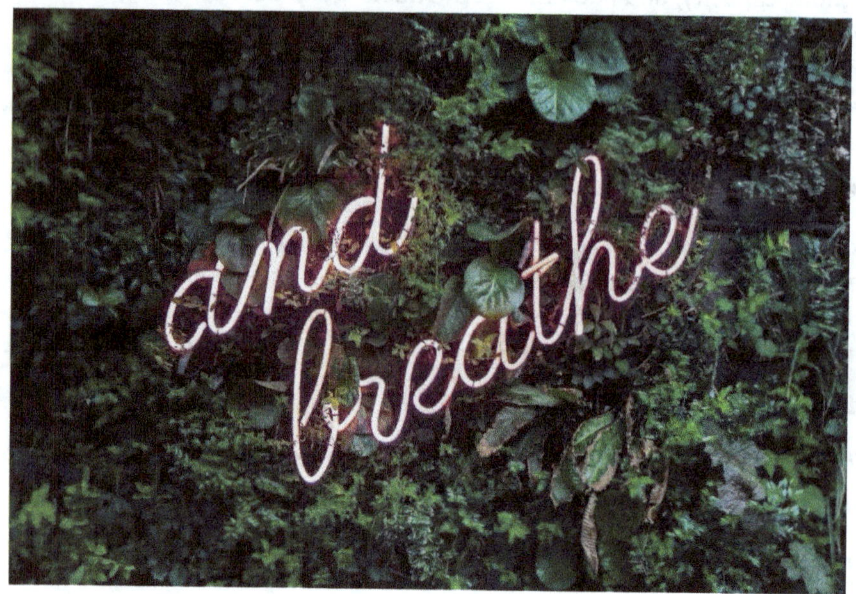

As I watched Antonia explain *nadi shodhana pranayama,* a yoga breathing exercise where one breathes through alternating nostrils by blocking the nares with thumb-pinky, I tried to imagine the physics of airflow through the nostrils and into the lungs. Breathing itself is obviously essential to life. However, most people think of breathing as just an oxygen delivery system, and do not give it a second thought.

Why does this work?

Why do people feel better after breathing?

Why do we need oxygen?

Why use those fingers?

While I stared at her amazingly cute dimples forming as she spoke, my brain wandered off into different things. However, she did give me a topic to write about later. Although yogis probably stumbled onto this simple technique that helped billions of people through thousands of years, the physiology and biophysics involved is pretty complicated.

And tedious.

And boring for most people.

However, if you're interested, feel free to read on!

Physiology of Breathing

Breathing is much like using a bellow (your diaphragm) that creates negative pressure that will pull air in. On a quick anatomy note; the diaphragm pulls air from the outside, which gets turbulent and warms up through your nose hairs and nasal conchae. Air then travels down through the trachea to the bronchi to the alveoli. The oxygen and carbon dioxide gets exchanged through the cell membrane into capillaries, which then carries oxygen via hemoglobin stored in red blood cells.

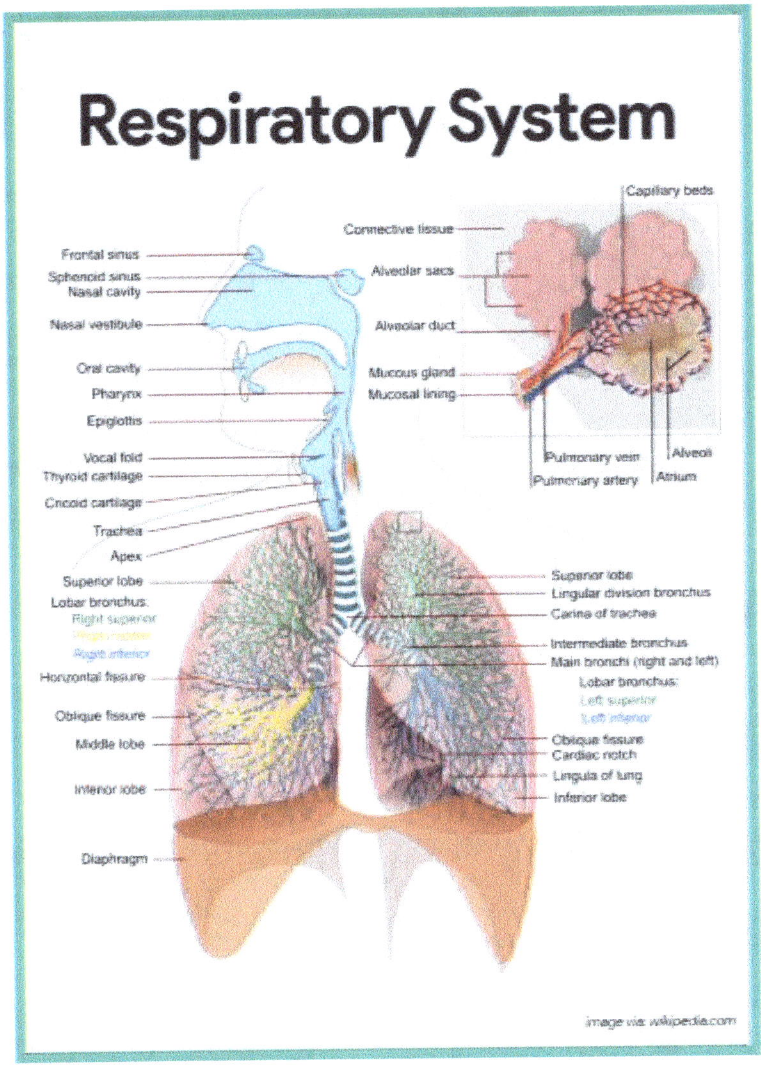

Carbon dioxide does some funky stuff via bicarbonate (acid), and with Le Chatelier's principle, gets pulled out of the bloodstream into the lungs. Carbon dioxide is then exhaled, and water is left over. When bicarbonate gets used up, it creates a less acidic (or basic or alkaline) environment.

Hemoglobin is amazing, and was one of the first few proteins ever studied. In acidic environments, hemoglobin will have a conformational change and release oxygen easier. In basic environments, it will attract and hold onto oxygen. This is due to the combination of the Bohr and Haldane effects.

That is why, in the few micrometers of space of the capillary that wraps itself around an alveolus, the carbon is exchanged out, creating a less acidic environment for the hemoglobin to catch oxygen downstream just before the red blood cell leaves the capillary and goes into an arteriole and eventually to areas that, through metabolic processes, release lactic acid, making an environment that creates a conformational change that releases oxygen from the hemoglobin grip.

Dammit, a run-on sentence.

The heart then pumps that red blood cell containing that hemoglobin around; and it goes through the cycle over and over again.

Amazing.

It is obviously more complicated than that. Bing Bohr and Haldane effects for more details.

Why Do We Even Need Oxygen?

Your body can make energy many ways. Aerobic (with oxygen) and anaerobic (without oxygen). To skip a LOT of details, your body runs mostly on ATP (adenosine triphosphate), a potent energy source that releases "energy" when a phosphate group gets taken off. Not important. ATP is created in many ways, but that is also not important. However, what is important is how the body converts sugar into ATP.

Anaerobic glycolysis (breaking down sugar without oxygen) ultimately only yields 2 ATP per molecule of glucose and creates a lot of lactate or lactic acid, which is the thing that burns your legs when you run a long time. Also, the same burning sensation of a heart attack; FYI.

When this happens, call your local EMS (194 in Croatia, 112 in the EU and 911 in the USA) immediately! Take 300 mg of Aspirin if you have it and sit or lie down.

This has been a PSA.

When oxygen is used, sugars like glucose goes into glycolysis and then into (tangent: WAY too many things to remember now and you will forget this, so I do not know why I am typing this) the tricarboxylic acid cycle. One product of the TCA cycle will then enter a process called oxidative phosphorylation, which through a series of electron transport chains that uses oxygen, phosphorylates (puts phosphate onto) ADP and turns it into ATP, and yields 30-32 ATP per molecule of glucose!

Carbon dioxide is a waste product of this process.

Bernoulli Effect of the Nostril.

Closing one nostril, which decreases the cross-section area of airflow, while keeping the same negative pressure from using the diaphragm in deep breathing, will increase the velocity of air going into the lungs, allowing more airflow pull from the outside to in. This is called the Bernoulli effect, or the same way you spray people with water from a hose in wet t-shirt contests.

When breathing out through one nostril, the increased velocity will create the same effect and a slight pull of air from the lungs, possibly getting rid of and circulating air in the dead space of the lung. Doing these exercises the recommended 2-3 times a day actually has the same effect as deep breathing methods, allowing a slightly higher concentration of oxygen to come into the lungs, while expelling carbon dioxide and possibly other micro-particles.

Not to complicate things further; there is always leftover air in the lungs that keeps it from collapsing, this air is like a room without a draft (*propuh* in Croatian). Without adequate circulation, it remains stale and usually smells of cigarettes. Long slow breathing clears out stagnant air that shallow normal breathing does not. That is why it is good to exercise to clear out pathogens, and that is why most athletes or people who regularly exercise for 45ish minutes a day (running, biking, etc.) do not have asthma or bronchitis.

Air out your dead space!

Have a pro position on the pro-propuh proposition!

Effects on the Brain?

Not going into that much detail, there have been many fMRI scans of brain function during yoga breathing or meditation exercises and the activation of different parts of the brain. In most cases, the brain releases dopamine (happy), cortisol (decrease stress), norepinephrine (or adrenalin; which also opens up airways), and activates centers of the periaqueductal grey area (endogenous opioid pain relief). This activation is also seen in many controlled breathing exercises, such as the Wim Hof method.

Wim Hof is a man famous for being able to control his body's reaction to extreme cold conditions and keep his body surface temperature normal despite being submerged in crazy cold water. By priming his body with his mind, the "fight or flight" response is turned on, which increases his body temperature and turns on all the areas of the brain that yoga breathing and meditation does. Except that he figured it out in Holland by jumping into a lake.

Relaxation Breathing and Diving

However, Wim Hof warns that his method should not be used before diving. In the good old days, divers used to hyperventilate before free-diving. Why was hyperventilation SO wrong? The Bohr effect. That would increase pH. This creates the more basic environment, and hemoglobin will have a stronger bond to oxygen. Oxygen will not be released in muscles (heart is a muscle). This will also cause vasoconstriction to the brain and other areas, thus causing the diver to have dizziness and eventually black out.

These days, relaxation breathing is practiced by competitive free-divers. Much like *nadi shodhana pranayama*, long slow breaths actually allow the maximum amount of oxygen to be in the body before making their dive. Since most people I know are not free-diving, their brains, which will get the majority of blood flow, benefit from the extra oxygen. Since I was an long-distance runner, I was also coached to have long slow breaths (8 steps in, 4 steps out). Thus, I would get more oxygen to my muscles and reduce the amount of lactic acid output.

Well, What Do I Know?

When my mentor at KBC Zagreb (REBRO) told me to do a lecture on Venturi masks, which limit airflow using the Bernoulli Effect (misnomer of the product, because it is not due to the Venturi effect; scientists are silly), I proved him wrong by saying that the central breathing center does not turn off when you give 100% oxygen, because a person in chronic acidosis will not stop breathing because of temporary alkalosis.

Removing more carbon dioxide from the circulation and adding more concentrated oxygen, the capillaries in the alveoli will vasoconstrict and cut off blood supply to that alveolus. The red blood cell cannot get to the alveolus, making no perfusion of oxygen and onto hemoglobin. This causes the person to stop breathing and, well … stop breathing.

He told me, while I was doing my lecture, that I was wrong. I told him that I was a biochemist and knew how physiology works. He told me to, "stop thinking like a biochemist and start thinking like a doctor."

I replied, "Doctors are only the bartenders serving the *beer* that biochemists create."

So, take a breath. Or a few. That was a lot of information for something we all do automatically, but we can control to make ourselves better.

Oh yeah. Why Those Fingers? Apparently, they are the pressure points for the sinus. Two birds, one stone.

I love those cute dimples.

She never called me back.

Pain in Your Brain Making You Insane? TRAIN!

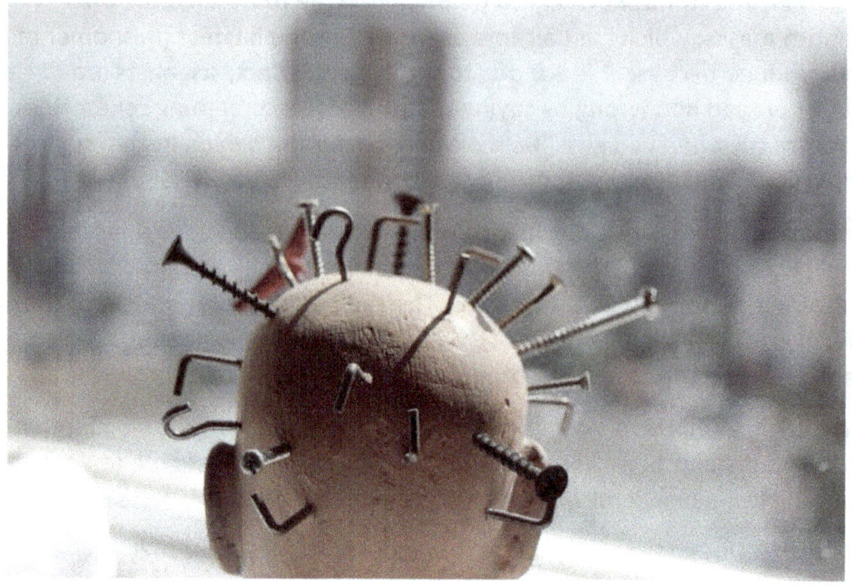

Why is getting kicked in the balls worse than pregnancy pain? After a few years, you do not hear guys saying, "Well, I wouldn't mind getting kicked in the balls again..."

Pain is one of the most difficult "symptoms" to deal with in medicine. I did not really believe the range of pain until I started working in the field and seeing people's different responses to pain; from kids writhing in pain even before I touch them to a man not even flinching when I debrided his wound. There are many examples in between where people range from yelling to a simple ow (in Croatian this is translated into "*ajoj*"). For a medical doctor, the extent of diagnostics depends heavily on "guessing" how the patient's pain translates into symptom or a real diagnosis.

For me, life cannot be without pain. For example, people feel angina pectoris from a stressful breakup to actually having dying cells from myocardial ischemia (heart attacks). I am constantly in "some kind of pain". So why do people feel pain differently? Nobody knows. There are many types of pain ranging from somatic, visceral, psychosomatic and central.

Putting aside all the medical terminology, these are pains that you feel depending on location. If you cut yourself, for instance, you will feel a sharp type of pain. If you notice, your pain will dull with time, despite the cut being there. Itching for some is sometimes painful for others. The diagnosis of pain is a difficult one and as doctors, we are trained to use the worst diagnostic tool (besides the Bristol Stool Chart) to gauge the value of pain that the person experiences.

Pain, being the main symptom of most patients, is then a very confusing symptom to deal with. What is important for us to know are the details of pain and that is done through **SOCRATES** (I am sure your doctor has asked you at least some of these questions to narrow down their differential diagnosis).

SOCRATES stands for: Site, Onset, Character, Radiation, Associations, Timing, Exacerbating factors, and Severity. Some pain symptoms, no matter the severity, is pathognomonic for certain diseases (i.e., RUQ pain radiating to back is indicative of acute pancreatitis).

There's a cheat sheet.

Don't think we're all clever.

Due to the controversy on the news about opioids (a type of pain medication) being over-prescribed for **CHRONIC** pain management, I would like to talk about that here. What is chronic pain? What are the different types of pain medication and what do they do? How do you deal with that pain? These are all hard questions and pain research, like most medical research, is relatively young. However, since pain is subjective, it is ethically hard to figure out how to research what pain really is.

For instance, a woman giving birth and tearing her perineum would rate a bad smiley face on the Wong-Baker pain scale; whereas a yuppie who had a silver-spoon life would cry at a papercut (not stereotyping, these were patients I have had). Even if you try to measure biochemical reactions of pain neurotransmitters while unethically inflicting pain on your subjects, you would get zig-zag, scatter-type graphs, despite trying to compensate for genetics, culture, gender, age, etc. Therefore, pain is a *VERY* open field and is still trying to be understood.

What Is Chronic Pain?

That is like asking, "What is pain?" Chronic pain is some sort of, usually and hopefully, dull pain that effects a certain region of your body or even sometimes your entire body. The latter is harder to figure out, but usually goes away with massages and feel-good activities.

However, most of these patients are in the older population, usually have had some sort of injury or surgery, and are prescribed opioids to manage their pain. Yes, that might seem like the lazy thing to do, but a doctor cannot manage a person's life as much as they would like to. On top of that, people really do not like following advice until they get scared with death (one of the side-effects of opioids).

That said, and in my field of rural emergency, I encounter many patients who are chronically on opioids, and get called for intervention because of diffuse chronic pain. It is a frustrating aspect of my job, where the only thing I can do is alleviate the acute symptomatic flare with more painkillers.

I will not go into the details of why someone might have chronic pain, but it is usually mismanaged. So how do we stop this? First, we must understand how we prevent pain, and before we do that, we must understand the source of the pain in the first place. So basically secondly, we must understand how we can prevent pain. So negatively firstly ... never mind.

So yes, pain. **SOCRATES**.

With **SOCRATES**, you can *PROBABLY* figure out why the patient is in chronic pain. What does chronic pain mean to you? Does that mean that you are incapacitated? Can you do normal functions at home? If you are hindered due to painful events, it does make life difficult and can cause stressful situations at home and at work.

That annoying pain that you have had due to twisting your knee when you were 21 can suddenly become debilitating when you are 35. Does that mean you are unhealthy and need some sort of medical intervention? All these questions on pain are related to the most important, and most forgotten, part of modern medicine; which is **QUALITY OF LIFE**.

If you cannot maintain your quality of life, then you are basically not fulfilling the WHO definition of health (physical, mental and social health). When this happens, it causes stress within yourself and your surrounding community. So how do most people alleviate that? Through taking prescription pills. Remember how doctors have thousands of patients and will say?

"Take this for a few weeks, please exercise [insert part of body here] and follow healthy habits and come back for a checkup."

Most people do not live a healthy life, which could exacerbate pain (sedentary lifestyles make some chronic pain worse). Some people must get back to work and physically do repetitive movements, which is the cause of the pain in the first place (please lift with your legs!). Like I said, most doctors do not have time to mediate lifestyles, so this is up to the population to understand and compensate. If I were a mechanic, I can fix your brakes and tell you not to brake so suddenly and plan your driving route. However, you probably would go back to habit and drive like a maniac.

If you do not want to be stuck on opioids, lifestyle changes are the key to chronic pain management. Since every case is different and every person has their own subjective opinions on pain, it is hard to say what the best course of action is. However, if you want your quality of life back and realize that even opioids are not working for you, then it is time to try different variations of pain management which does not require addictive medication.

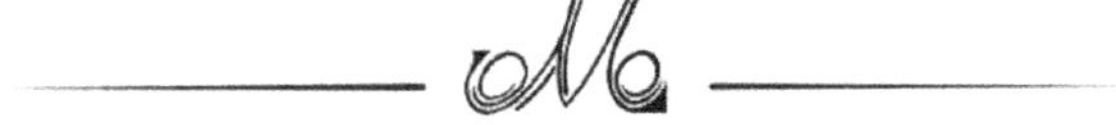

The Good Stuff?

In a few quick paragraphs, I would like to delve into some commonly used painkillers, and quickly describe what they are generally good for. You can research these online to see what works for different occasions, but everyone reacts differently to pain medication because nobody knows where their pain is coming from. To understand the type of pain, you have to understand what alleviates it.

Aspirin

Aspirin is described as a near-perfect drug. Being used for a LONG time in its "alternative medicine" form as a hot drink to relieve fevers, the base of aspirin is (you can just Wikipedia this instead of me writing out a synopsis) an anti-inflammatory and a COX inhibitor.

Long story short, this type of inhibition blocks the interleukins (biochemical messengers) that cause pain and fevers. Besides being bad for your stomach by not blocking acidity production and protection thus causing ulcers, there are few other side-effects (super fever by taking too much). This universal painkiller is good for headaches, muscular cramping and joint pain.

Acetaminophen

Another commonly used pain killer is APAP (paracetamol, Panadol, Tylenol or acetaminophen). Found through a fluke, APAP is amazing at cutting off pain and is still poorly understood. It has a COX2 inhibiting property, which makes it act like aspirin in a more specific way and reduces fever, but it is also somewhat bad for your liver (do not take with alcohol!), since it is metabolized in it. There is also a mechanism where it blocks pain transduction in the spine itself, so it is very good for peripheral pain symptoms that are not due to inflammatory effects (sprained ankles and such).

This painkiller is combined with other potent painkillers to create combinations for "hard or heavy" pain, which is taken chronically and can cause potential liver problems later in the future. I would use APAP for fevers and not chronically, although it does help.

Ibuprofen and Other NSAIDs

NSAID stands for Non-Steroidal Anti-Inflammatory Drugs. From the name and a little bit of logical medical knowledge, you can derive what it does. There are MANY drugs in this category and they all do the same thing to different levels of relief. Since they are an anti-inflammatory, they can reduce immune reactions in your body, creating a range of relief from the inflammatory reactions that cause arthritis to the inflammatory reactions that cause fevers.

In that sense, they are good when your joints are inflamed when you twist them or injure them in any way. Since they work on different places of pain management, I like to alternate NSAIDs and APAPs daily to effectively reduce ACUTE symptomatic pain.

Opioids

Despite being the derivatives of heroin, modern biochemistry and chemistry have honed their art to making key-lock mechanisms for the super-addictive nature of the natural painkiller, opium. Basically, working on natural opioid receptors, these natural painkillers will block almost most types of pain. Unfortunately, they are still very addictive and if used chronically, they will cause upregulation of the receptors and you will need a larger dose to get the same level of relief.

Most chronic pain patients are treated with opioids and thus the controversy in modern medicine. Although prescribed to alleviate pain during physiotherapy, most patients will subconsciously feel pain after and discontinue their physiotherapy in lieu of a quicker pain fix. Dr. House?

The Chronic!

When I was training for triathlons, people would tell me to get high so that I could lift weights better. I was not a smoker so it really irritated me, but I could tell you that it worked. I could hardly feel pain for the few hours that I was high, but that comes with any downer high (like opioids). Since medical marijuana became a "thing", many chronic pain patients are on the chronic (and many more who are not in pain).

The Mary has potentially decreased the amount of productivity in the working class, so I will not talk about this further due to a lot of conflict from recreational users, who could alternatively be sipping willow bark tea (aspirin) to lower their pain levels, advocating the "goodness" of a "natural" drug that has some mental side effects.

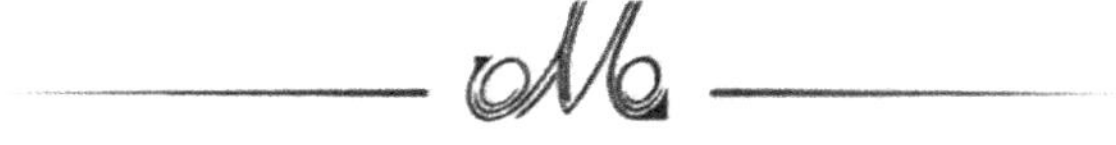

The Alternative? Better Than Drugs?

So why do not we just alternate drugs and treat CHRONIC pain through mixing pills? Well, it's complicated. If I was not there to regulate, would you really comply? Honestly, would you? And the second is that chronic pain is different. Once you start taking pills for years, your body will eventually get used to the pills (will NOT explain upregulation, Bing it). Is there a better way? You bet there is! What is the alternative?

You will not like it, but the healthier option is (obviously) a healthy lifestyle. That might be a vague concept, but chronic pain disappears when you are in a state of less stress. Imagine chronic muscle pain and then getting a massage. Imagine your boo-boo when you scrape your knee and your mother blows on it. Imagine your back pain when you are having amazing sex.

Yes. All these things block pain receptors in much the same way that pharmaceuticals block them and if you want to know the biochemistry and physiology behind it, feel free to use Bing. Reading chronic pain management articles on the inter-web from variable sources, I based it on **T.R.A.I.N.**

Nooo!

Train

You have to exercise. You must regulate your body to stretch your muscles and increase circulation. Most people will feel pain in the beginning and it will be overbearing, but after a few weeks, your body will compensate and down-regulate those pain receptors and you be able to manage the symptom of pain.

Rest

The body needs to regulate itself and most people are in the constant state of bad stress. When you do not get enough bed rest, your body will always be in the state of shock and stress causes pain (again with the biochemistry). Meditating on the pain can also alleviate the pain and, done properly, it can also relax the part of the body disturbing you.

Antioxidants

Besides stopping smoking and drinking (which most patients will not do), antioxidants will combat these toxins that you are putting in your body every day. If you follow any type of nutrition website, anything can be an antioxidant, but try to include potent antioxidants. By creating a protective barrier against oxidizing stress on your body, you can better alleviate symptoms due to (well…) smoking and drinking and other social determinants of health.

Information

This might be the most important aspect of medicine that people seem to forget. Trust your doctors, but always question their decisions. Be well informed on how to increase your quality of life and the more you share with your primary physician, the more they are informed on how to manage your lifestyle so that you can further improve your condition and not rely on heavy medication to alleviate your pain.

No!

"Just say no!" was the 1990s anti-drug campaign I grew up with. These medications are made to alleviate pain while you recover and not to keep you in a constant state of addiction. During a CNN interview, a 65-year-old man had to go to rehabilitation to treat his oxycodone (opioid) addiction, which was prescribed to him to deal with his chronic pain.

Sometimes, you have to say *no* to your physician, and better inform them of what you are dealing with. After all, it is your health and your **QUALITY OF LIFE**.

Or occasionally get a COX block.

Anti-Aging: A Hot Button Issue

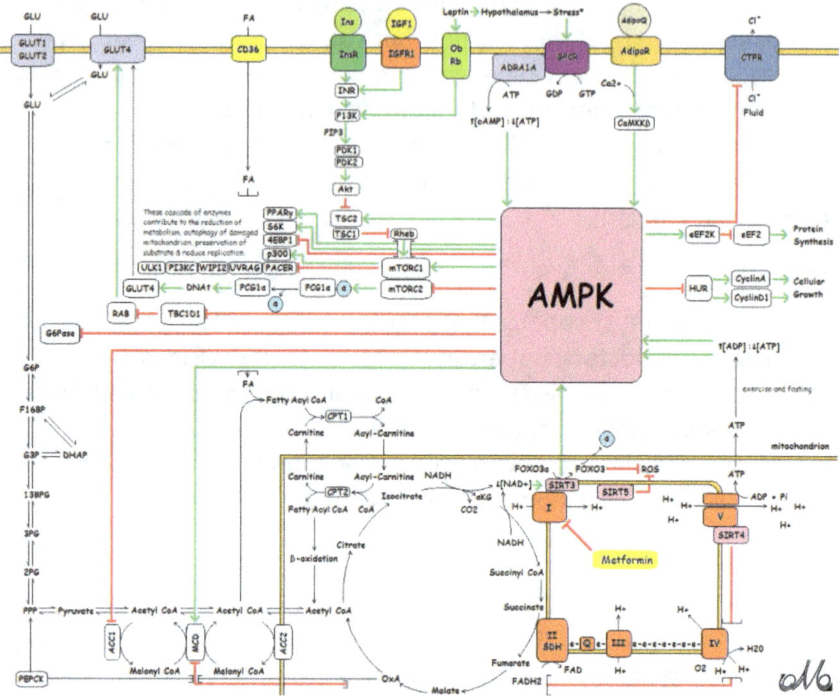

Metformin's mechanism of action. This figure also generally explains where anti-oxidants work, how prolonged exercise reduces fat and what that does to your metabolism, how intermittent fasting works, primary diabetes mellitus pathway and some treatment options, what happens when you eat glucose or fat, where cellular aging is regulated, and some basic metabolic pathways.

A new entry into the ICD-11 (international code of diseases) is aging. Thought of as a natural process of all living things, the WHO has taken a step forward in adding 'aging' (MG2A) into the newly released ICD-11 list. Seeing a natural process as a disease is a big psychological step into realizing that researchers can treat aging as an amendable problem; by either increasing lifespan, remedying quality of life, or by finding solutions to reverse the process.

Although very few researchers are in the field of aging, there have been steps into understanding the processes of cell death and cell regeneration, due to the popularity of cancer research and gene therapies. Understanding the causes that trigger cell death and cell regeneration, aging can potentially be slowed and hypothetically reversed. There are several specific pathways being studied in cell apoptosis and cancer research, which range from regulating mTOR (mechanistic target of rapamycin) kinase to gene therapies that reverse muscle cell aging in mice.

Only a few medications can be considered as the holy grail in pharmaceuticals. The closest to date is aspirin, which has a few side effects that can be addressed by literally sugar coating the problem. Other than that, aspirin has multiple benefits with very little side effect.

Metformin is starting to be the other. Besides being very affordable, metformin is a staple medication in a DMII (Type 2 Diabetes Mellitus) by regulating gluconeogenesis in the liver and increasing target cell insulin sensitivity. This is done through downstream cascading effects when metformin binds to and down-regulates MCI (mitochondrial complex I). These newly understood "side effects" of metformin could be potentially beneficial in anti-aging research.

Unlike other single-shot techniques in addressing the problem of aging, metformin has a shotgun effect on the cellular aging process. By suppressing MCI, metformin mimics fasting and stress responses to the cell. By blocking the usage of metabolic substrates, individual cells respond by slowing replication and cellular metabolism.

This has a few desirable effects that are beneficial to both anti-cancer and anti-aging research. By mimicking a stress response, cells are signaled to pause replication, induce autophagy of damaged mitochondrion, remove and fix ROS (reactive oxygen species) damage of DNA, and reverse metabolic processes to increase energy stores for "better times".

Other *obvious* downstream effects of metformin are reducing glucose levels by increasing insulin sensitivity through the IIS (insulin/insulin-like growth factor signaling) pathway, increasing uptake of glucose through GLUT4 expression, and reducing oxidative stress through decreasing excessive ROS in the mitochondria. These effects are the main reasons of using metformin since the 1950s for DMII.

Paradoxically, metformin, through suppressing oxidative phosphorylation, promotes other complex reactions that can increase intracellular ROS that signals activation of the SKN-1 (skinhead 1) / Nrf (NF-E2-related factor) pathway, which is cellular protective; at least in C. elegans. In addition to improving other cellular functions, SKN-1:

1. increases cellular stress response, which is known to increase life expectancy in the same way intermittent fasting does,

2. detoxifies and thus being expressed especially in the gut,

3. balances redox by reducing ROS,

4. increasing lipid metabolism and thus increasing mitochondrial function,

5. increases immune responses,

6. and signals the build of collagen and extracellular matrices.

Metformin indirectly regulates the SIRT3 (sirtuin 3) pathway, which maintains mitochondrial mass and bioenergetics by acetylizing mitochondrial proteins. This regulates certain genes, such as VNTR (variable number tandem repeat) alleles, which is closely related to cellular aging. SIRT3 also binds to SHMT2 (serine hydroxymethyltransferase 2) and upregulates one-carbon metabolism during glucose starvation of the cell. SHMT2 is in the series of enzymes of the mitochondria that can also reduce redox stress by using ROS to metabolize single carbon substrates into purines. On top of that, SIRT3 upregulates mitochondrial DNA replication and transcription in chondrocytes, increases antioxidant reactions in endothelial cells, and is a regulator for mitochondrial biogenesis.

Due to mimicking fasting or exercise, metformin has also to increases the intracellular ADP to ATP ratio, which activates the AMPK (AMP-activated protein kinase) enzyme. Exercise – and other cellular stresses such as intermittent fasting – is more potent at activating AMPK through usage of ATP. In stressful situations, hormones from the hypothalamus can activate G-protein coupled receptors, which releases cAMP as a secondary messenger.

The correct concentration ratios of cAMP:ATP signals the cellular stress response, which activates AMPK and regulates the series of enzymes to stimulate glucose uptake, free fatty acid oxidation, and decrease synthesis of proteins and lipids. However, cAMP – in an over-abundant concentration – with PKA (protein kinase A) is a signal for cellular apoptosis. AMPK suppresses mTOR kinase, an enzyme that blocks mitochondrial autophagy, increases protein synthesis, and induces cellular replication in response to insulin.

Mitochondrial and general cellular activity declines with age due to ROS damage, and/or mutations in the DNA. Although AMPK has been observed to be involved in the regulation of healthy mitochondrial function through mitophagy and upregulation of mitochondrial biogenesis, the sensitivity to AMPK also decreases with time. Therefore, AMPK activators, such as metformin (and exercise, and intermittent fasting), are currently peaking interest in the research community, since they not only potentially extend cellular life, but also maintain cellular health.

Interestingly, aspirin seems to improve metformin function by augmenting the AMPK enzyme by phosphorylation of AMPK at a different site (Thy-172) than PKA (Ser-485), thus increasing the activity of AMPK. Phosphorylation of Ser-485 adversely effects metformin's effects by inhibition of AMPK and subsequently increasing gluconeogenesis by hepatocytes. However, phosphorylating Thy-172 with salicylate, AMPK activity enhances metformin's role in suppressing glucose production, thus increasing the effectiveness even further in terms of mediating DMII, and potentially aging.

As a biochemist turned medical doctor, understanding processes at a protein level is crucial to understanding the natural process of a disease. By understanding nature's technology that took billions of years to produce, researchers can always find newer technologies that are viable for the population to increase quantity, and most importantly, quality of life.

Analogous to life – in all its research and understanding – any processes and function comes down to two variables: **concentration** and **time**. Understanding that, any disease – even aging – can be understood and eventually reversed.

Mental Health

Everything is Binary | No Gray Areas in Life | Lifestyle of a Libra

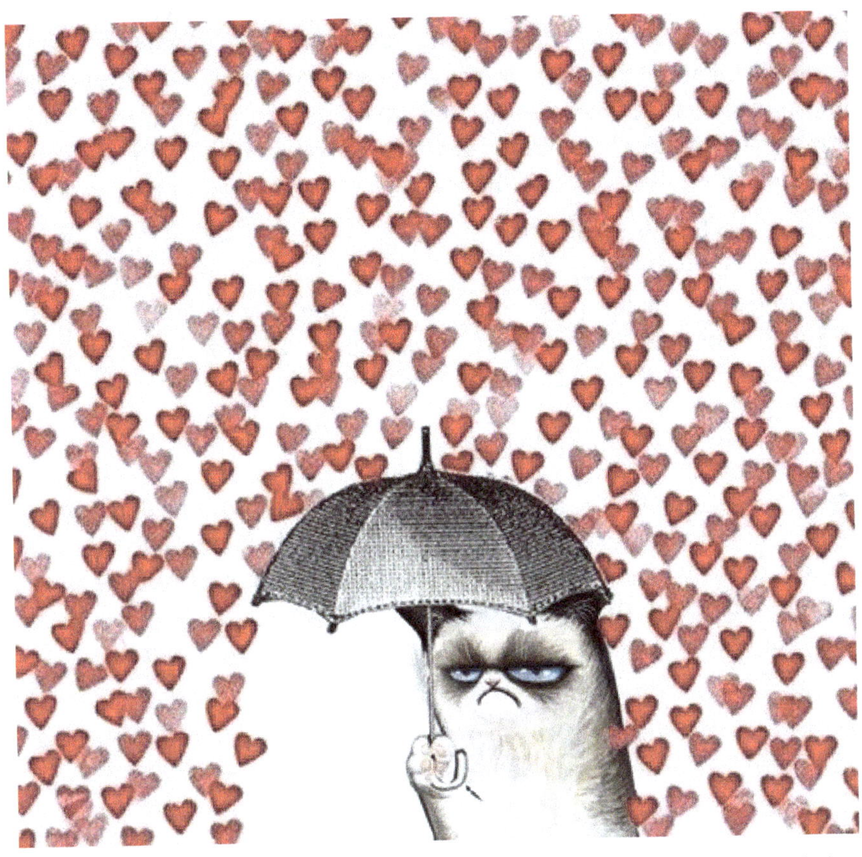

It's all about balance. I can only tell you my story, because everybody has their own sad story. Their own cross to bear. Their country song to sing. I do not believe that most people are happy, because depression and anxiety is a global pandemic that everybody has struggled with at least once in their lives.

Major depressive disorder (MDD) is a result of anxiety gone wrong; a complete imbalance of neurotransmitters. How does this happen? The mechanisms to understand the imbalances are simple. However, to fix the problem requires a lot of work, self-reflection and acceptance.

Trauma is one of the common factors fueling anxiety, and eventually depression. Although on different ends of the neurotransmitter spectrum, one influences the other. That is why psychiatrists like to put people on a regimen of Rivotril and Fevarin; or whatever SSRI and anxiolytic of choice that the pharmaceutical companies "persuade" them to prescribe. This chemically balances the neurotransmitters enough for a patient to listen, comprehend, accept the situation, and create new synapses or habits. In addition to drugging the patient, rebalance is accomplished with a LOT of psychotherapy, which does not happen in social healthcare systems.

I grew up in a happy childhood. It had its traumas, but nothing that was life-changing, because I could logically explain things. That is until I came to Croatia. I then realized that my life was not logically explained, but was dictated by emotions of others, which was not very logical. My tasks or chores would be either be completed, or be delayed depending on if the person got laid or not. Obviously, that is a joke because making that statement MIGHT offend Croatians.

However, living in Croatia, every action was a lottery. Nothing could be planned. Emotions effecting people's ability to do their jobs, and comprehensively judging others, has affected me from passing classes in medical school, to getting a stay permit in Croatia to continuing university. I will not even mention decisions based on skin color encountered in the 21st century.

This to me was not logical. This to me was and is still my trauma. This led to my anxiety. That led to my depression.

I sought out psychiatrists, was on Rivotril and Fevarin, went to counseling with Gestalt psychologists, and tried cognitive behavioral therapy when I turned to social determinants of health. CBT did not work, because apparently this type of behavior is acceptable in this culture. This is where I am now. For me to start something takes a LOT of determination and energy. Accomplishing something brings me no "Aha!" effect or joy. So why does this happen? How did my happy brain get to this point?

Being a medical doctor and biochemist, I'll tell you how I got this way, and possibly how to fix it.

As many of you probably read, the brain remains plastic for your entire life. Forty years ago, people thought that the brain settled after the childhood plasticity phase, but that has proven to be wrong. The brain is able to create new neurons (neurogenesis) and create new connections (synaptogenesis). This is the cause of creating new habits, new skills, and new beliefs. On the other end of the spectrum; trauma, anxiety and eventually depression.

Danijel Dubičanac of Hatha Yoga Croatia then asked me to read into Yoga. I have my opinions on Yoga in the "West", but will keep them to myself at this point. However, there is no harm to question why a few-millennia-old tradition and lifestyle have worked for so long. Why does MDD happen mostly in Western nations, and less in Eastern nations that follow similar rituals of Ayurvedic or other Eastern cultural lifestyles?

Ignoring the other lifestyle habits of Ayurveda, Yoga seems to be the most adopted Eastern "habit" in the West. Doing Yoga regularly seems to "balance" people. There are people on both left and right of the normal distribution, but on average, Yogites are less anxious, less depressed, and more balanced individuals. I have met MANY "outliers" though. So as a quick review to doing Yoga, which is similar to Islamic prayers and Tai Chi and other Eastern lifestyle habits, there are five (four) major points of Yoga that share similarities to those other lifestyles:

*Proper exercise (**āsana**)*

*Proper breathing (**prāṇāyāma**)*

*Proper relaxation (**śavāsana**)*

*Proper diet and positive thinking (**vedānta**)*

*Meditation (**dhyāna**)*

I do not want to go into detail into *WHY* these Yoga points are beneficial, nor compare Ayurveda to other lifestyle choices, because the result is basically the same (despite people fighting over these beliefs): the balance of neurotransmitters and the creation of good habits.

There are a lot of studies done with EEGs, fMRIs, rats, cadavers, and biochemistries that show benefits of Yoga (you can Bing medical articles on your own time), but any regular exercise will have the same end result. The problem in MDD is to get motivated and get started.

Depression and anxiety are often classed and treated together as synergic diseases, like chlamydia and gonorrhea. If you have one, you are bound to have the other. Logically, if you are constantly anxious, this will inhibit your ability to live life normally, and that will eventually lead to depression. On the other hand, when you are depressed and are not living your life normally, you will be anxious around normal things. Thus, the goal is to balance the neurotransmitters that are either too excitatory (anxiety) or too inhibitory (depression).

The major players of excitatory neurotransmitters are monoaminergic neurotransmitters, which many non-pharmacological nutritionists try to upsell, are dopamine, serotonin, and epinephrine. Most people try to increase these neurotransmitters by taking supplements and believing that you are what you eat (vedānta). However, the small effects of dietary supplements are not enough to reduce the symptoms of major depression, which not only lacks neurotransmitters or receptors, but also is due to the increase in inhibitory neurotransmitters. This is the general idea, but it obviously gets more complicated.

In "newer" studies, MDD has also been linked to LOW GABA levels. Despite being an inhibitory neurotransmitter, GABA has different receptors that can negate a negating synapse. As the brain has billions of neurons with an infinite number of connections, there is no way to isolate depression and anxiety into a few simple pathways. Thus, the working theory is a disbalance of excitatory and inhibitory (E/I) neurotransmitters.

In the prefrontal cortex (PFC), GABA neurons control the E/I balance as well as the excitatory output to projecting areas; such as the amygdala, bed nucleus of stria terminalis, and the dorsal raphe nucleus. The complex network of GABA neuronal connections from the PFC to these other areas of the brain are important in mediating complex emotional and cognitive processes in the brain. Both are important in anxiety and depression, and the irrational decisions made while in the state of depression (and other sociopathic states).

When both monoaminergic and GABA neurotransmitters are either low or high (or disbalanced), this causes changes in emotions and mood. Although this could be normal, large emotional changes, such as trauma, can leave a longer-lasting, stronger "negative" synapse. This will cause an imbalanced pathway that needs to be corrected by either neurogenesis or synaptogenesis, and the only way to do this is to train your brain over time.

This is where Yoga comes in handy, both as preventive medicine and a treatment option.

A few studies have been done that measured EEGs, which show higher alpha and theta waves, which correspond with lower anxiety and stress. Theta waves are also associated with information processing and alertness. Looking at neurotransmitters, a study showed that GABA levels have also increased after regular Yoga sessions. After 12 weeks of Yoga, subjects claim to be less depressed and anxious compared to a control group.

Yoga also increases production of monoamines, especially serotonin and dopamine, causing relaxation and reward. Combining the explanation from above, Yoga potentially improves MDD and anxiety by effecting the E/I neuronal networks from the PFC by balancing out the GABA and monoamine neural pathways.

People know that Yoga works. But why? So far, everything has been an educated guess (like most of neuroscience). Reading through research papers and picking out more plausible explanations, I can briefly explain why the five points of Yoga works to improve symptoms (without writing an entire PhD thesis about it, and not getting a PhD in Alternative Medicine).

Āsana

Posture and positioning are important in muscle control, strengthening nerve endings, and is commonly used in physical therapy. As an ex-wrestler (or anybody studying martial arts), perfect moves and practicing perfect posture create muscle control that gives you an advantage over your opponent. This increases circulation to the muscles, and leads to generally better health.

Like Islamic prayers, having certain postures creates "goals" of movement, and the feeling of "something that you need to do". That necessity counteracts the negative neuronal networks of depression, although it could exacerbate anxiety by creating necessities.

Prāṇāyāma

The act of controlled breathing has been discussed enough to scare away a Yogite I went on a date with. These are the people I stay away from, because despite listening to her gospel of pranayama, she practices Yoga without adopting any other part of the Ayurvedic lifestyle.

In short, controlled breathing decreases acidity in the body, and glutamate could potentially be turned into GABA by a shift in concentrations (Le Chatelier's Principle).

Śavāsana

Before anxiety starts, proper relaxation NEEDS to be taught and practiced. I currently live in Croatia and coming from the USA, I realize that not many Croatians know how to relax properly. In fact, nobody knows how to relax at all; not at work, not at home, and not even on vacations in their coastal weekend houses.

MOST CROATIANS I KNOW OWN COASTAL WEEKEND HOUSES AND USUALLY AN ORCHARD OR A VINEYARD!

Why are they not smiling!?

A colleague said it the best when he said that he rather vacation away from Europe, because when he has to go to the coast, he ends up having to clean the coastal house, cook because restaurants are too expensive, and spend thousands of Kuna driving and paying for tolls. His vacation is just bringing chores from his home in Zagreb to his vacation house on the coast.

Whereas, with the same amount of money spent to go to Hvar from Zagreb by car and staying there for a week, you can fly to Malaysia and stay in a resort on the beach, eating in restaurants and not having to worry about cleaning, feeding or the unnecessary responsibilities of life. Life in Croatia has been overly complicated for me, from dealing with racism to unnecessary bureaucracy. After a vacation, I need a vacation.

Since the pay is so low here and the prices are more expensive than East Coast USA, I use my vacation to save money instead of spending money to pay for gas to get to work to earn money to pay for gas to get to work. This causes anxiety and that led to my depression, as my vacations are spent in my living room, unable to afford any form of eustress.

Vedānta

The power of positive thought is one of the most important tools for treating depression. CBT and sometimes hypnosis is used in psychiatry to seed positive thoughts and habits into an individual. Positivity is self-explanatory; that creating a belief of goodness will reaffirm the rewarding dopaminergic neural pathway.

An excess of excitatory neurotransmitters in this area without balance of the E/I neurotransmitters from the PFC might cause a manic behavior, and when those neurotransmitters are exhausted, a person can sink into depression. Positive thoughts, and proper diet in a distraught environment not only balances out the internal self, but also the outer social aspects if most people in society are this way.

Dhyāna

Meditation relates to positive thinking with a mantra. There are many meditative techniques (not just Ayurvedic Yoga) and depending on the culture, meditation can consist of clearing thoughts to accepting all thoughts and "releasing them" by acceptance. When a person thinks enough on a subject matter, the brain can come up with solutions to the problems. Two brains are better than one. Three are better that two. Social interactions can also be a form of meditation, and group meditation can increase social awareness.

Meditation can then contribute to combating depression and anxiety by balancing mood and behavior; and most importantly, acknowledgement and acceptance by the society that the person is in. Meditation can also put logic to traumatic situations, which the binary brain needs to process the uncertain and troublesome situation.

Should you Yoga?

Therefore, it does not really matter what you do to manage MDD and anxiety. You can be a Cali girl and do Yoga in petroleum-based yoga pants and think you are saving the world (*OMG!*), or you can be a devout Muslim ritually praying five times a day.

The point is to create a stable belief system that will rewire your brain to accept the faults of life, and create a regular habit that promotes better behavior. Anxiety and depression lie in the gray areas of uncertainty. In order to believe and accept, you must choose. Negative or positive. Black or white. Or to be a little less racist-sounding; brown or browner.

Do not forget the mantra of **B**ELIEF, **A**CCEPTANCE AND **R**EGULARITY!

Or **B.A.R.**, where I have been going to deal with my own personal depression.

:-/

Knowledge Yields Empathy

Empathy begets knowledge.

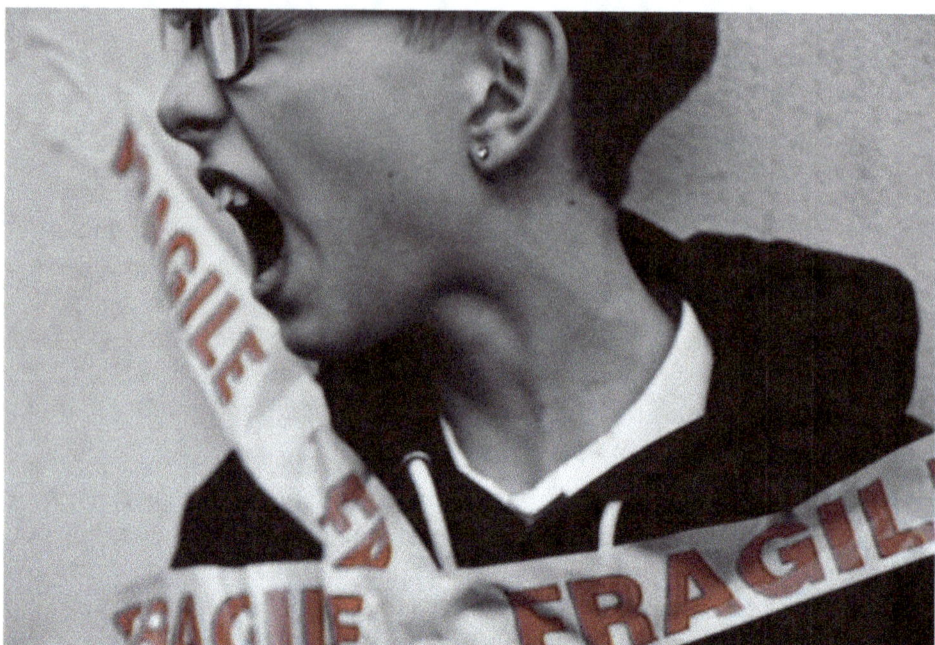

I drive the car looking out for motorcycles, because I ride a motorbike. I ride the motorbike looking out for cyclists, because I also ride a bicycle. I ride my bicycle looking out for pedestrians, because I also walk. I walk as if any two-ton vehicle is out to kill me. I ride my bicycle as if any two-ton vehicle is about to hit me. I ride the motorbike as if any two-ton vehicle is about to crash into me. I drive the car as if I have been handed a shotgun.

Take this as an analogy to life. People with power need to empathize with the people who are not blessed with it. People who are not blessed need to be wary of the people that can ruin their lives at their own whims. This is an ugly world that we live in, because the top percent cannot empathize with the bottom percentages. They have never been in those positions, so they drive in their two-ton killing machines as if they are the only ones on the road.

As I drive through the streets and highways of Malaysia, I – myself – get furious at peoples' lack of consideration and illogical mindset, and end up verbally **SCREAMING** my internal thoughts. People who know me will think I am impatient. People who do not will think I am mentally deranged.

I would curse God and attempt to get an answer as to why God created these idiots if perfection was well within the realm of possibility. Even given free-will and choice, God can easily influence our minds into a better choice, either immediately or through the Rube Goldberg series of events that led to that person cutting me off in their motorbike; forcing me to slam on the brakes, so I do not kill a person with my two-ton vehicle. If those series of events did not happen, people around me would not think of me as mentally deranged.

Someone can advise me that "the buck stops here," and that I should be the one to stop this cycle of anger and frustration. However, these crazy events happen too often that they themselves become the norm. I am also not alone in my reaction. People have reacted worse than I have, which have resulted in physical manifestations of anger.

We are then labeled as crazy, anxious, impatient and bipolar. We are the ones who need to be medicated with anti-anxiety medications to be able to suppress the fact that others are the cause of our reactions. In my own cognitive behavioral therapy, my psychologist told me that I am normal in an abnormal space. I can explain my actions logically, but most people that I talk to, who cause potential harm to themselves and others, have the same answers:

"I do not know."

"Because I felt like it."

Why do we have to suppress our logical norms in order to appease the whims of the status quo? Should the status quo not empower themselves with logic – and knowledge and empathy – so that they do not put themselves in danger; either by getting hit by a vehicle, or a person who manifests their anger with a baseball bat? When this happens, the authorities in power are quick to blame the driver of the vehicle, stating that we should have a sense of R.A.D.A.R. in our brains or a form of natural *echolocation, so that we are constantly aware of our surroundings.*

As Mental Health Awareness Month comes to a close, I hope that people took the time to empower themselves with knowledge. The height of my anger and external outburst – which in Islamic religions would put me in Hell – is analogous to the explainable reactions of the people in society who are labeled for having different mental capabilities. In Croatia, people who study mental "illnesses" are "defectologists". As if these people were "defects" compared to what people perceive as a normal society; those "normals" who weave in and out of traffic without care for themselves or others.

Normal is relative to society and time. There are many cultures who base their societies on religions, and still hold social injustices as normal. There are more cultures who base their norms on skin pigmentation. Not many cultures base themselves on logic and evidence, because if they did, the population would be in charge, instead of the top aristocratic percentage holding power.

The world needs empowerment and empathy, combined, to understand the people who have been blessed to be born outside of what society calls "normal". Anybody who has an outburst – or sink into themselves, or have separated thoughts that help them survive in an oppressive society – most often have a reasonable reason to their current condition. These people should not easily be labeled as manic, depressive, nor schizophrenic.

They are mostly misunderstood by societies' lack of knowledge, their laziness to understand, and the "I want it now" attitude of medicating the outliers until they comply to the normal curve of that society. If mental differences are illnesses, why do not they also condemn people who have obesity, diabetes, heart disease or cancer?

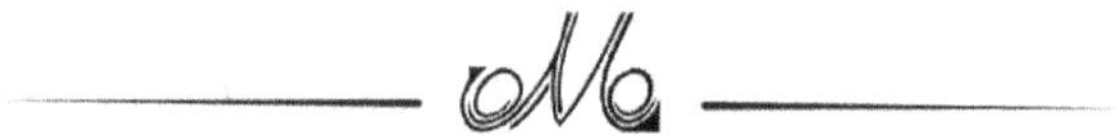

Mental Health Awareness Month is there, not for the status quo to gawk at and sympathize with the HUMAN BEINGS who are outside of their societal bell curve, but it is there as an opportunity to empower people to understand that they ARE human beings. There were events that promoted artists who are labeled as autistic (introverted), and promotions of help for people who are going through rough patches (emotional) – usually due to the lack of acknowledgement and empathy – in their lives.

I hope you went to those events to get empowered, and I hope that it sticks in your brain cells so that you become part of a society who understands the outliers; expanding the standard deviation of your own populations. I hope you take the time to understand these people and their thought processes, include them into your society, so they themselves become the norm.

Unfortunately, like the goldfish people are, once the marketing of these Awareness Months is over, most status quo will revert and ignore these people, get angry at them, and eventually add them to the list of problems plaguing their society. These HUMANS will be medicated and suppressed, so the status quo would not have to spend their time to understand and incorporate them into their twisted version of humanity … until the next Mental Health Awareness Month.

Help people become people, and not just shove them aside until next year. Accept people as people so that these "Months" become a daily norm.

I Ergasia Fernei Vasana

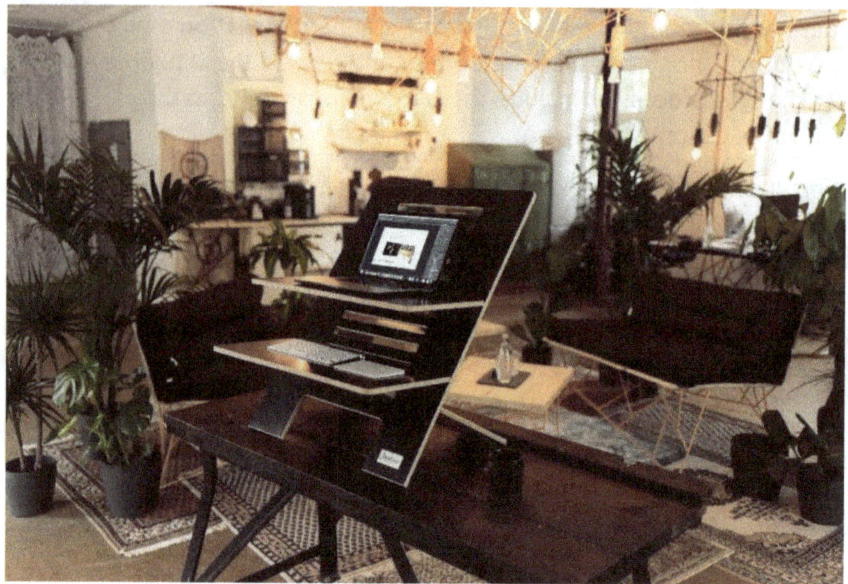

Most people would prefer quality over quantity; except for employers screening resumes for total number of years worked. My superiors, of every department I have worked in, often come to me and see me lounging, waiting for the next patient or call for a field intervention. Then they would proceed to assume that I am not doing work.

They are right. I am not working. Because I am lazy.

That is my **strength**.

I am lazy, but I am also obsessive-compulsive. I need things to work logically; not just in my own brain, but in the surrounding environment affecting me. Therefore, I would spend sleepless nights **automating** everything, so that I can be found lounging on the couch with nothing to do. When I am found doing nothing, that means everything is automated.

Working in Emergency Medicine, we always have to be ready. We must limit our biomechanical movements, so we can be fast. That requires efficiency of the workspace, which a lot of employers have not begun to consider when designing an office space. Of my many elective psychology courses, **Ergonomics** was one of those semesters at NC State that opened a whole new world for me. I was not born with skills of organization. I was taught and nurtured into being organized and efficient, so that my goal of ultimate laziness can be achieved.

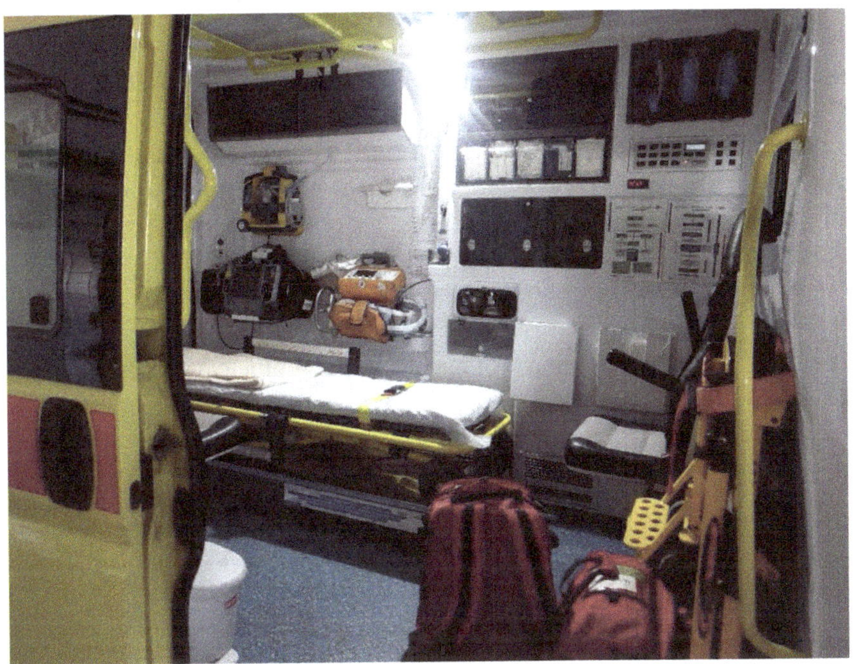

My office.

A doctor and a nurse can work with minimal movement. Everything is organized from head to toe and from most critical to least critical emergencies. The bags are organized to first have access to equipment that measure vitals, then open up into airway, breathing, circulation and then drugs. Medication is not organized alphabetically, but by conditions and by head to toe. This way, name changes or changes to pharmaceutical company contracts do not interfere with the organizational ergonomics.

Any doctor can come in and quickly comprehend the ABCDs of emergency medicine, and even though that doctor does not know what medications the clinic has, they can see what we have available for the condition they diagnose.

Ergonomics is using logic to organize. Organization leads to fewer mistakes. This is VERY important when you are in Emergency Medicine.

Ergonomists and behavioral psychologists are employed by bigger firms to minimize stress to the employees; whilst yielding the highest output of quality and quantity to their customers. **This reduces stress on everybody**. Since people spend more than a third of their lives in a modern form of the production line, efficiency of that system could lead to a better quality of life for the individual; whether you are the server or being served.

Due to false marketing, the majority of people relate ergonomics only to furniture or electrical input devices (keyboards and mice), not knowing that it is also a psychological concept designed to make our lives easier, physically, mentally and consequentially socially. Asking a few people in Malaysia, the concept of ergonomics is stuck on implementing only furniture design to decrease stress on biomechanics. However, the other sides of ergonomics not only allow the prevention of long-term physical injuries, but also allows an increase of efficiency and quality of the workplace through improving biological and psychological inputs and outputs.

Ergonomics, according to the APA Dictionary of Psychology, is "the discipline that applies a knowledge of human abilities and limitations drawn from physiology, biomechanics, anthropometry, and other areas to the design of systems, equipment, and processes for safe and efficient performance."

Since ergonomics falls in the realm of psychology, psychological understanding of culture and society play an important role in creating effective work places, reducing stress and ultimately increasing health indexes, where an employer can realize that the same output can be done in a fraction of the time. This can reduce the number of effective hours worked, but sadly, due the nature of human selfishness, profit will most likely be prioritized by the employers, leading to no changes in the health statuses of their employees.

In the 21ˢᵗ century, there is no need for the antiquated nine-to-five (plus overtime without pay in most cases) if the quota of the day (or week, or month) have been met. By prioritizing profits over the health of the employees, employers and their companies have ironically decreased the quality of output by burning out their workers. **Burnout** (F43.0 in ICD-10) is a common and serious condition that not only affects performance at work, but burnout can trickle down to other aspects of the employees' lives, negatively affecting family and social dynamics, promote substance-abuse, and further decreasing employees' work output.

Burnout due to work stress is a common cause of social tensions, post-traumatic stress disorder, domestic violence, or simply major depression. These issues, commonly seen in family clinics, are seemingly without a known "cause"; since distress at work is accepted as being normal for current and older generations.

Due to lack of recognition and empathy, need for profitable output, and the power-hungry effect of *"dollar dollar bills, ya'll"*, employers will eventually lose trained and experienced individuals. They are then being replaced by workers who need to be retrained for positions; ultimately using precious time and company resources. Employees, who are more appreciated and acknowledged, tend to be more committed to the company. However, these days, people are not treated as people or valuable company assets, but more as disposable cogs.

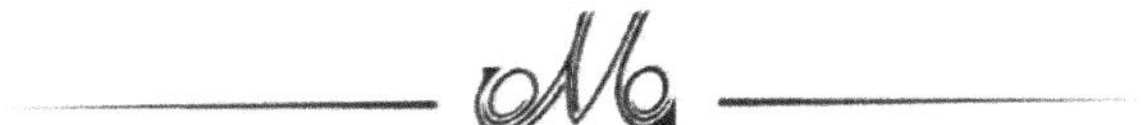

Preventive medicine is always the best medicine, so to prevent burnout at work, employers can implement simple (and cheap) ergonomic designs and psychological steps to increase the quality of life for their employees; who then do not have to come to me with sob stories that I have to medicate with anti-depressants and benzodiazepines.

Comfortable chairs and safety equipment are necessary (but costly) to decrease the mental stress and physical stresses of the worker. Cost is usually why most employers do not spend their profits to protect their employees. However, providing personnel with proper personal protective products, work injuries – such as postural injury, repetitive strain injury, carpal tunnel, vibration syndrome, etc. – can be avoided, and experienced employees can endure employment and evolve efficiency.

Adjustable 'ergonomic' furniture protects and promotes good biomechanics. These ergonomic solutions protect the body by avoiding unnecessary strain. However, if the workflow is efficient enough, people can take regular pauses that reduce health problems by breaking stagnation. This reduces the need to spend monies for ergonomic products.

Efficiency of the workspace is not just limited to biomechanics. Organization and order of inputs can maximize the efficiency of output. In my line of work, equipment must be bedside ready, organized from more urgent to less urgent, and organized in accordance to importance of the ABCD (Airway, Breathing, Circulation, Disability) order in Advanced Life Support. This theme is repeated for all our supplies and equipment.

There is an inner ring closest to the patient that can support the patient in very emergency situations (crash cart, monitoring equipment, medications and an anaphylactic kit). The middle ring is for less emergency situations (gauze, splints, sutures and other trauma equipment). The outer ring holds non-emergency items such as our primary care medications, extra supplies and storage area. Medications are organized into emergency cases, and then into physiological systems from head to toe.

This might seem logical, common sense and intuitive. However, before my arrival, the clinic was organized haphazardly. There was no dedicated crash cart, the oxygen was in the storage room and not ready bedside, the medications were organized alphabetically by brand name, and everything was stored by the organizational method of "where can I find room for…"

The computer was turned to the side, so that doctors would have to turn their backs to the patient while typing their report. Having to listen to a patient and create rapport by personal contact, this type of setup doubles the time and allows mistakes in dictation, as the doctor would have to turn and type what they remember after listening to the patient.

Considering multiple doctors work in the same space, medication and equipment were hard to find, and that lead to time being lost during emergency situations. Having no crash cart meant that the team had to get individual equipment together, often from the ambulance, to even start reanimating. This can lose precious minutes that directly effects the chances of patient survival.

By ergonomically organizing the clinic, treatment can be started immediately, and this contributed to our department's successes in reanimation, our speed in diagnosing, and successfully treating patients. Since clinics were standardized, anybody who worked in other outpatient clinics could come to any other clinic within our Department of Emergency Medicine, and immediately recognize the setup and know where things were kept. Emergency ambulance bags were standardized and organized in the same ABCD theme, so doctors and nurses did not have to waste time to review the entire clinic to orient themselves.

Offices can be organized the same way in the order of importance; most used to the least used. This allows the employee to save wasted time, and react quicker in obtaining materials needed for work. If the work is static (at a desk or standing in one spot), the most useful items would be placed be at an arm's length, ideally organized by systemic function of the job itself.

Alphabetical organization might be easy to implement, but it requires unnecessary thought and movement when searching for a commonly used item. Organization by usefulness to the organizer (this happens a lot in professional kitchens) would be useless to another worker. In my job, organization is patient-centric. In other jobs, organization can be centered around the main output, whether it be burgers or printouts. The flow of inputs is then organized with any bottlenecks at the start, so that the flow of output matches or exceeds the input.

In addition to the biomechanical aspect of ergonomics, there is also a psychological component that can be utilized to enhance the efficiency of work spaces by decreasing stress or increasing productivity of employees. Besides being the calming color of trees in nature, **green** reduces strain on the nervous system by reducing strain on the eyes. This is because the cones of the eye perceive green wavelengths (550 nm) better than other wavelengths. Green is taken advantage of in places where people need to be calmed, such as hospitals.

Personally, I have not seen many office spaces utilizing green colors, or even better, a green mural of nature. Alternatively, indoor plants have a better effect on decreasing the stress level of employees, so that work output is more efficient.

On the other hand, these psychological tricks are also usually played on customers and the general public.

Ergonomics extend to **GUIs** for operating systems and phone applications. **Placement** of products can be used to keep people in the stores (or malls or casinos). Supermarkets used to have a combined entrance and exit, and separation of the two physically forces customers to walk through the market, signaling a sensation to buy. **Signs** are optimized and used to efficiently direct people into or out of places (airports or hospitals). Different **Colors** are used to get attention, either for advertising or for people's safety (red as warning, yellow as changes, orange as hazards, blue uniforms for acceptance, green exit signs for calm, etc.). McDonald's has changed their signature yellow and red to more earth tones, making subconscious suggestions using the natural color of cooked food (in addition to the smell). **Cookies** or cookie sprays are used by real estate agents to signify the concept of home.

Without full knowledge of these psychological tricks and analyzing the motives of corporations and government, it is not very surprising how humans have **very** little freedom of choice, and easily succumb to the illusion of it.

Do you naturally close your OS windows on the left or right? The psychology of ergonomics can change human behavior in less than a decade with clever marketing. Most people cannot even imagine a life without "smart" devices, and we have arrived to the generation of newborns who are born with one.

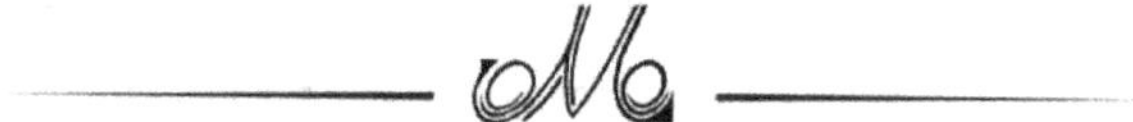

To protect the population from trauma, stress and burnout, work spaces can easily be reorganized in a weekend, and can be constantly evolved to create a safer workspace; both biomechanically and mentally. Implementing green (and sometimes baby blue) is one of the cheaper methods for offices to protect employees from constant burnout. Plants are also a cheap option, and some plants clean stagnant office air and require minimal care.

There is minimal cost to reorganize a work space for efficiency, and time can be saved, as well as, employees can be protected from biomechanical and mental injury. Kuala Lumpur ranks third in the world for most-overworked city. Employers need to realize that - by not implementing alternatives to our outdated work ethic - they **DIRECTLY** affect the health of the population by increasing physical and mental stresses from burnout, and taking away valuable social time from friends and family.

Make things better.

Every work space is different, psychology and common sense is cultural, and it is difficult for me to explain logic in a simple sense to a population that does not analyze and appreciate the larger picture. Most people spend more than 33% of their lives at work and commuting, and this problem is bigger than just reorganizing office space. It affects generations of brainwashed individuals into thinking that work brings happiness by obtaining temporary materialisms that temporarily increase dopamine release.

The structural ladder of societies and outdated city plans in current metropolises have led to the system we have now, and it will take more than just office planning to obtain work efficiency and optimum health of the population. Government implementation of laws to protect its citizens will be lobbied against by profit-hungry corporations.

The overall goal, which today's outdated mentality still ignores, is to increase the quality of life for everyone in each population. That way, we are not stuck in the age of industrialism, and can finally move to the 21st century.

Braining Too Quickly

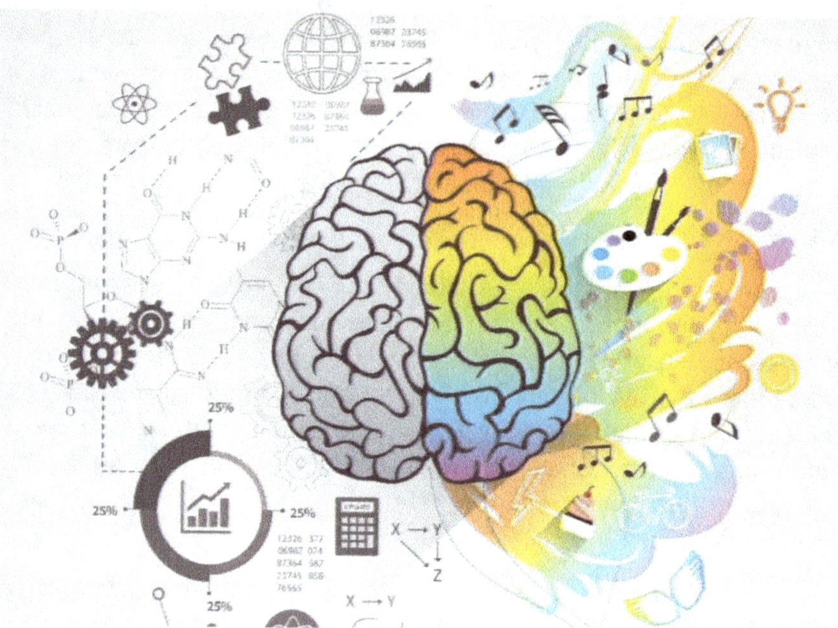

Designed by macrovector | Freepik

I do not like to ever call the lighter spectrum of mental "disorders" disorders. ADD (me), ADHD (me), light schizophrenia (me), and autism (me) are some of the disorders that I have dealt with almost on a daily basis (patients). People come to me because of "frustration" (anger) or "depression" (sad), which are just different results of the same trigger. It usually takes me a few examinations to understand their triggers.

I am in primary care (emergency, family, general medicine), so people come to me first. I would write my report that either a psychiatrist or a psychologist can refer to. Obviously, I cannot get to the root of their issues after a 15-minute conversation, because people usually avoid their personal weaknesses (honesty counts!) when they talk.

I would guide the conversation to their social lives, and how they react to their surroundings to get a better sense of how they think. At that point, I am not necessarily trying to find what their triggers are. That would take a long time. I hope the psychiatrist can find those triggers, and sometimes they do, and that is the first step of self-realization.

In Croatia, I can send people to free consultations with centralized hospitals. They can go private, but that is expensive for most people and more difficult, because people with depression symptoms are usually unmotivated. I know I was, but I had friends who would be there for moral support, sit in the waiting room, and wait for the consultation to finish.

I work in rural areas and villages far from any tertiary support, so it is hard to motivate my patients to go for a 1.5-hour ride (even though I can offer free transportation for them) to the hospital, waste the whole day, and then get back to their villages. I am surprised that they even come to see me, because most of them are from satellite villages.

Back to ADHD.

Basically, I was lucky to be "diagnosed" early, so my teachers and mentors knew how to guide me. I was also lucky to go to private schools (where teachers were not paid peanuts, and actually care about one-on-one student interactions), and to NC State (where class sizes were small and there's a big emphasis in finding students who show promise). I also met a lot of friends who acknowledged my natural, random curiosity and - unlike my parents - did not yell at me or use the rattan.

ADHD is not just a psychological disorder. There is a big neurological component to ADHD, which involves general changes in the gray matter. Although gray matter size is seemingly smaller, the gray matter density is higher, creating closer connections (possibly more connections). The brain is working "faster" by utilizing the more available connections. Gray matter is responsible for cognitive thinking, but some hyperactivity of the gray matter can be debilitating when cognitive decision-making skills are constantly being bombarded with different choices.

That is why amphetamines work. They activate the neurons in the neuronal connections that suppress overactive neurons. They also activate neurons that give the "feel good" dopamine feedback, so people feel satisfied long enough to not jump themes.

Personally, I think that some of these newer "diagnoses" should not hinder our mentalities. The natural behavior of overly active individuals is very influenced by social "norms". Society only works on a narrow band of the normal distribution of behaviors. Depending on culture, behavioral norms are usually skewed. Most people who are considered "not normal" by society are not normal, because they are outside the two standard deviations of normal societal thinking. However, what is "normal" for most people?

Most of the time, it is because society, friends and family (and most people) are not patient enough or interested enough to listen and understand. They are quick to judge and are prejudiced to people outside of their small bubble of "normality".

My adopted brother's behavior constantly angered my parents, and he eventually got diagnosed and medicated for ADHD. My parents wanted him to become an Imam (Islamic version of a priest). They sent him to religious schooling, which he did not enjoy, and rebelled against. He was then labeled as stupid and had anger management issues. He was constantly yelled at throughout his childhood for being forced into a hole that his peg did not match.

Now at 20, he stays in his room with minimal interaction with family. If parents and educators just took time to nurture his interests (FPS games at this time), his entire personality would have been different. There would be a positive reinforcement structure instead of a negative punishment for not meeting societal and cultural criteria.

I know this, because I have been through it. I only found myself when I left my family's and culture's social and religious "structure". I was able to explore other venues when I was out of local society. My parents would ask me if that is how my friends communicate to their parents, because I would argue with them (much like my adopted brother).

I said, "YES!"

It was not about the arguments, but it was about challenging their views with **facts**.

I grew up with multi-cultural friends in the USA whose parents would listen to them, respect their opinions, guide them, and usually adjust behavior and habits based on logic. It was much more nurturing, and I started to become a cultural chameleon. I thought it was OK to have an opinion. However, when I came back to Malaysia, it was very not OK.

People who question religion were considered "free thinkers". Some friends actually asked me, "Do you want to think freely?" I just stare at them to see if they can catch their own Freudian slip, but they do not. To me, it was not very logical to not think freely, because the opposite of free thinkers would be mental prisoners.

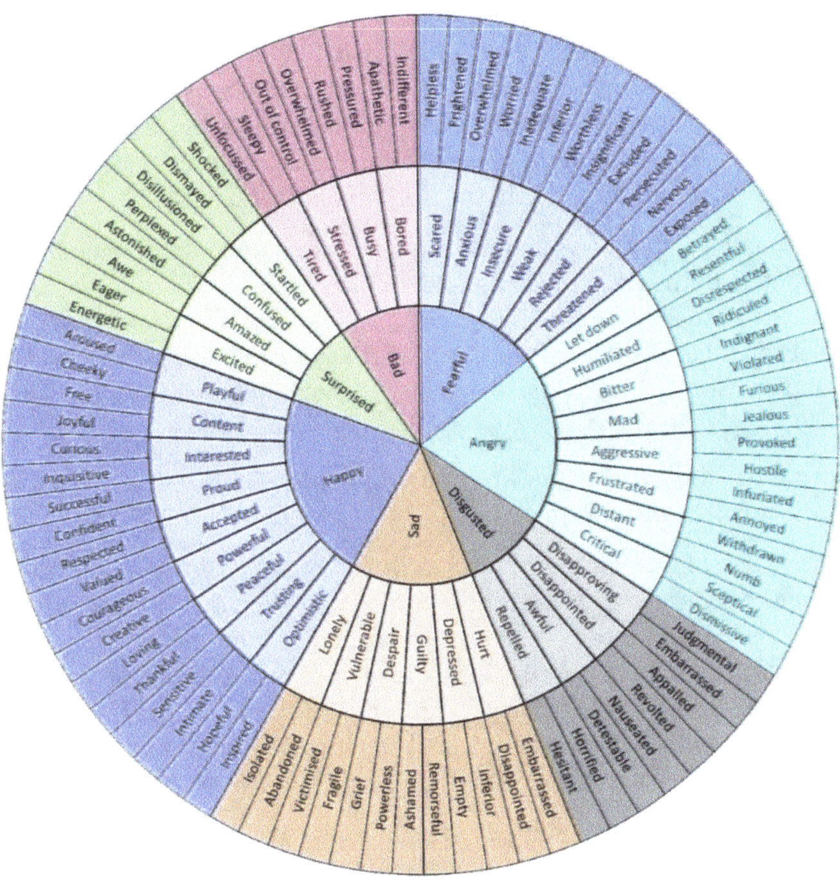

Created by Robert Plutchik.

Get to Know How You Really Feel

There are 7 basic emotions. Depression is a deeper stage of sadness, and has changes in neuronal connections. That is why medications are needed, and a lot of additional therapy (or just talking) is needed to reestablish logic. A lot of "why" questions must be asked to recreate structural logic in the brain.

This works, because brains remain plastic until you die. Just depends on how much and how long you want to train your brain (we all get lazy). Some AI work is helping understanding synapse rewiring. Luckily nature does it automatically through synaptogenesis.

ADHD can be a root trigger of depression. Just because society is not patient enough to handle your exquisite neuronal connections, society and culture are quick to label with a DSM-5 diagnosis. Autism is (almost) the same way. Yes, they are over-introverted, but I have seen autistic kids and adults snap into communication once they find the right trigger: music, art, etc. They will be completely "normal" within those interests. Their close influences can then guide them to use their personal experiences of "art" to relate to the environment around them.

Unfortunately, it is **always** about the relative viewpoint and normal distribution of the (local) societies. ADHD (and persons with other mental "changes") usually do not fit into society, and most outcasts easily fall into anxiety and depression. Frustration (anger) takes over, and eventually disappointment in society could paralyze you with depression.

You probably do not have depression. You are saddened. You are exceptional in a "normal" society, and you are alone because very few people can keep up with you.

This, of course, took me a long time to write. For the past weeks, my brain has been distracted, and that is normal for many people. Not many people can concentrate fully when they are surrounded by the constant and useless stresses of normal life. A friend once said, "Don't worry about doing it. Once you feel like doing it, you'll do it well." There is a trait that most people with multiple centers of concentration have, and that is the ability to hyper-focus.

This might seem counter-intuitive to people with attention deficits, but that is probably because of the idea of multiple neuronal pathways overwhelming concentration. However, when these multiple pathways can separately concentrate on one theme, then we are able to focus the many facets of input (learning) and output (execution).

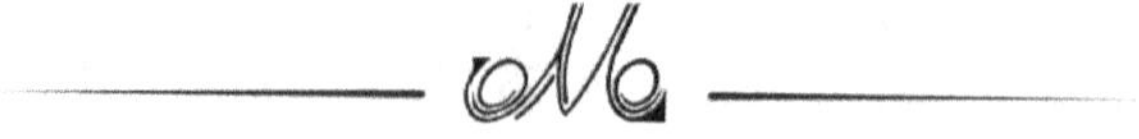

At 17, I did not understand chemistry until my mentor guided me to imagine everything in 3D space. I was stupid and dyslexic in 2D. I was hired to tutor kids for the American School in Zagreb who had "learning disabilities" and were diagnosed with ADHD. One teacher took a chance on me, and I tutored one kid and brought his grades up from D's to having a 3.2 GPA in his senior year. How? I played basketball and just injected information by saying, "Did you know…"

We did more than basketball. We went for drives, walked through forests, talked over drinks, etc. I was tasked to just tutor him in biology, chemistry and math, but ended up teaching him to think and use his "weakness" as his strength. I got paid a lot to do that, because tutoring one-on-one is a personalized, life-lasting education. Why can't most parents learn about their kid's "disorder", and guide kids themselves?

Modern society seems to dump problems on others instead of having a culture of DIY.

Simple Habits to Make Yourself Smarter

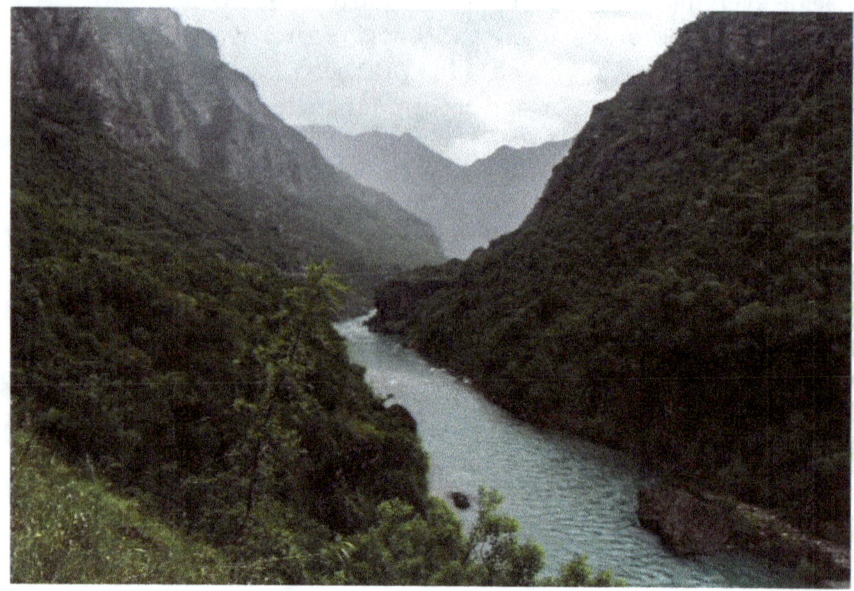

Can you make yourself smarter? The answer is yes. Fifty years ago, people have thought that the brain cemented after growth and old dogs cannot learn new tricks, but through research in synaptogenesis, the brain is a lot more plastic than originally thought.

Working as a medical doctor and through interaction with a wide array of people, I realize that most people are not as smart as they think they are and limit themselves to one facet of interest in their lives. If they are farmers, they would know things about what they are farming and nothing else. Most of us drive, but we know nothing about how to fix a car.

The brain is the most complicated part of the human body that has more connections (synapses) than there are visible stars in the sky. However, did you know you have more than one brain? The intestinal tract itself has its own network of synapses, and it is connected to your brain through slow hormonal messaging.

There is a brain "coach" on the inter-webs who charges over $1000 a course to take advantage of your brain functions; a course that can be summed up to **talking** to each other and **listening** to each other. To learn, you obviously need some basics. The learning curve is through repetition and after the first day of memorizing a fact, you will only remember around 97% of it. If you keep repeating it, you will remember around 70% of the fact after a week.

To skip paying more than $1000 for a three-day course, all you have to do is **talk** and **teach** those facts to others. When you teach, your brain repeats those facts, and when a conversation ensues, you will remember those facts due to the brain storing traumatic things better than they remember good things. Teaching is stressful. This is also why post-traumatic stress disorder (PTSD) occurs, but you cannot remember when you went to Disneyland and what you ate a few days ago.

This is probably why most girlfriends (at least those who I have dated) only remember that 0.0001% of something you did wrong and forget the majority of the times that made her happy. Then after years, she will use that one excuse you forgot to dump you.

:-(

The brain runs heavily on sugar and ketones. In fact, there are some studies that ketones reduce the risk of Alzheimer's. There is such a thing as the blood-brain barrier, and overdosing on vitamins, minerals and antioxidants are good for your body, but a waste of money for your brain.

The list of foods listed on the website of that online course is "good", but many people do not realize that most of these ingredients cost a lot of money if they are not local products. Stick to tomatoes, green leafy vegetables, less meat, less carbohydrates, and any fruits and vegetables.

A Croatian lady once asked, "If I took turmeric pills, will I live longer?"

My reply was, "Indians eat turmeric for breakfast, lunch and dinner. You are about 60 years behind in preventive medicine."

Note*: I got tired of writing about antioxidants, because everything seems to be one.*

Exercising is good for your body, and releases dopamine and natural opiates, which makes you feel better and feel less pain through older age. However, it does not significantly improve memory function, because concentration and cognitive repair comes from better sleep and recovery.

Depending on the type of person you are, negative comments can push you OR positive comments can push you. People have mostly told me that I could not do something, and that urged me to prove them wrong. When people give me positive comments, my brain stops motivation, because things are "good enough". These days, I ask myself, "How can things be better?" That way, things are never just "good enough".

Depending on your personality type, psychologists have changed classifications over time from "introvert and extrovert" to "type A to C", and now the popular "Jung and Briggs-Meyers". As long as you follow your type, you are able to utilize your brain to its maximum capacity.

Writing things down is a form or repetition. So is having a morning routine, or any form of routine. I used to work in Emergency Medicine for 10 years, where there was no routine at all. After half a year, I still cannot sleep, thus lacking the most important part of increasing brain capacity, cognitive function and learning capabilities.

Sleeping is the most important part of the day to let your brain reset. Nobody is an expert on sleep, because it is not well understood. Insomnia, or lack of sleep, can lead to symptoms ranging from narcolepsy to epileptic attacks. The current theory is that the brain reorganizes information and "toxins" are removed.

Having broken sleep will affect the brain's capability, which God should have known. Although - in Islam at least - building the modern prayer schedule around farmers and sheep herders, we now have light bulbs that ruin our natural sleep cycle thanks to Edison and Tesla and pressures from society to stay awake at night.

Regularly reading can also help cognitive function. This is not necessary if you need to speed read, which the "brain coach" teaches in a $1000 course. Most speed readers scan for information, instead of reading the book word-for-word. This is only useful if you are learning a new language. However, I do agree that scanning information improves your memory. It is like that game back in the day where you scan a picture for ten seconds, and write down the details of what you saw.

What games were I made to play during my childhood?!

In that sense, to improve brain function, sharing information, social interactions and teaching is the best way to go. I still remember the 99.99% (*max 90%*) of my relationships, because I repeat the "good".

Play a game with your friends.

Teach them a new fact.

Learn new things.

Let people complete sentences.

Do not just hear.

Listen.

Sleep.

In a Box

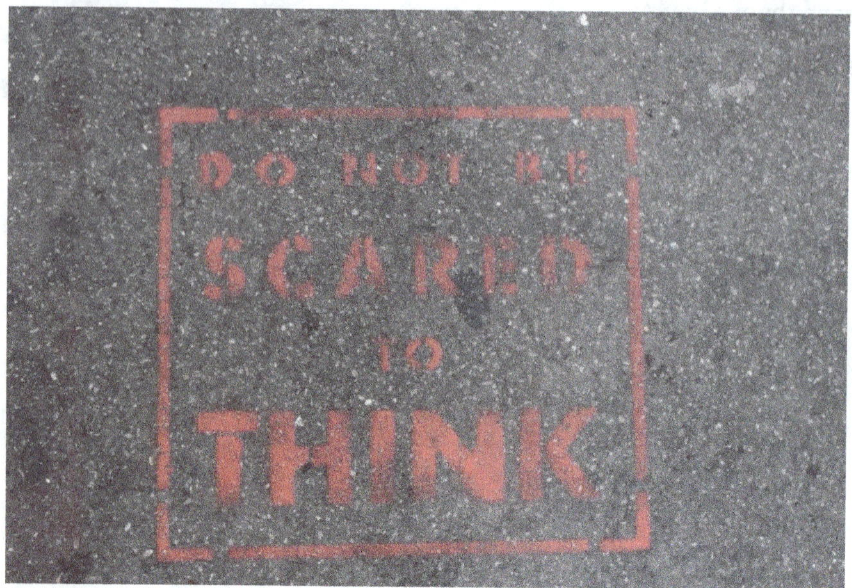

"Society is collapsing, and people are starting to recognize that the reason they feel like they're mentally ill is that they're living in a system that is not designed to suit the human spirit."

- Russell Brand

Most everyone in Croatia, who I have met, says the problem is me and not them; the culture, the society.

Instead of practicing tolerance, letting me be me and nurturing my skills, these people making up society impose their language, food and culture upon my already established personality. People are afraid of what I can do when I am let loose. Only in the USA did they let me loose, and at the age of 21, I made my pharma clinic almost 4x more profit; from 1.2 million dollars to 4-5 million dollars per month. That was after one month in the company. Just imagine how much further I could have gone if the economy didn't go to *$h!t* due to the attack on Wall Street.

Croatia held me back.

Everything I did to make every clinic at which I worked more ergonomic was met with criticism (even though they use it that way now, and even take credit for it). The concept of ergonomics is lost in Croatia, but it was a psychology course at NC State University. I did not grow into this naturally; I was taught how to think and to create an environment with the most efficacy.

Like most US universities, I went for one major and was allowed to (and encouraged to) explore outside my major. I took electives from psychology to cinematography to choir to orchestra. Even physical activity is encouraged in all majors, in which I did triathlon class and club, and outdoor survival training.

I could advance in classes, and followed my pace instead of being held back like in the Medical College at the University of Zagreb. Since the pace was slow, I could come in drunk, sleep through class, and still maintain a B average.

At NC State, I finished my biochemistry course load by end of 19-years-old (I entered university at 17) and was able to teach biochemistry to my peers as an undergraduate! I was one of two undergraduates advanced enough to be able to teach the course. The other was Bryan.

The sky was the limit! Until I encountered the Croatian culture, and was mentally bashed into subservience.

Malaysia, I am disappointed to say, does not work on innovation either. They earn money by selling raw resources, but not manipulating them. People are so comfortable here that they can concentrate on hedonism, and leave the responsibilities of the world to others.

Those others happen to be people like me.

Ego!

Social Health

Dulcius ex Asperis

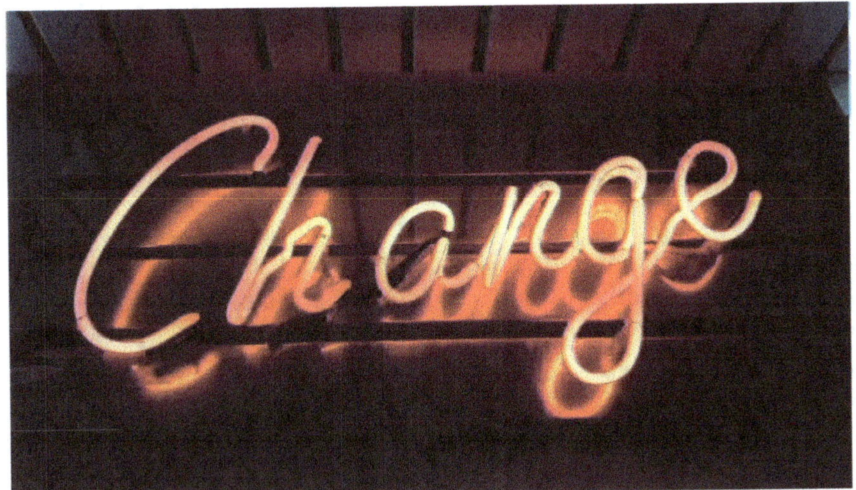

Despite what everybody thinks about health, it is not just **physical** well-being. Many governments, and people stuck in the status quo, regularly ignore **mental** (for some reason, is still taboo in the 21st century) and **social** (worsened by the social media technology in the 21st century) health.

Almost everybody lacks empathy. Those who do not are often misunderstood as being a pushover. Those pushovers are stepped on until they explode. Then they are often misunderstood for being crazy. They are medicated until they also lack empathy. We can all change this with a little acknowledgement.

I was having lunch with my doctor uncle and – in common Yeop-style – was ranting about the lack of innovation in this Malaysia.

He asked, "So why do not you innovate something?"

I replied, "What problem do you want me to fix?"

To which, the reply was crickets.

There are abundances of problems in this world that need to be addressed, but are we willing to find solutions to them? Or do we stand there with no thoughts nor ideas to contribute, and let crickets do the chirping?

As I sit in his sterile, first-class home, which has a roof and doors, and a Mercedes (among other cars) parked out front, I was not expecting any answer from this apparently redundant question. You cannot ask the status quo this question. There is no need to ask this, as people hardly empathize with someone who is at their lowest point. I have been in my uncle's position, and I have been in the opposite position. Believe you me, lowest can always get lower.

I have been homeless and left for dead. Not of my own volition, but of the whims of a government that would not let me work due to my citizenship. A piece of paper stood between homelessness and a position as a medical doctor. My qualifications did not matter; my experiences did not matter. Just a piece of paper stood in my way from eating trash to working and improving pre-hospital Emergency Medicine in almost every county I have worked in.

Unlike those who have not had the humble experience of homelessness, I do not like taking praise or credit, so I allow others to do so.

There are many problems that can be fixed in Malaysia (and most other nations) ranging from human rights issues to religious non-freedoms to governmental corruption. All of these can be found in many articles on Bing, which I will not even bother to list out. Being a Biochemist, most innovations and inventions that I am interested in usually happens in more advanced countries; Malaysia not being one of them.

I was informed that my cousin is working on stabilizing protein structures (I am assuming at higher temperatures), which has been done many times within the past 25 years through help of heat-shock proteins, or with the example of the new mRNA vaccine (spike proteins are proteins). There are many people working on this – I have read a lot of the research – so I am not sure which level my cousin is inserting their skillset into.

Yes. Innovations are hard, but they just require thought. Inventions are harder, because they require anticipation. Hardly anybody thinks that far ahead into the future to invent solutions to problems that have never existed. Most people today who innovate, tweak a product, and then claim it as theirs. Therefore, most "ground-breaking" innovators are there to just "manage symptoms" of the issues we are facing today.

For a superficial and redundant example; do we really need a better cellphone? Do we need this step-by-step approach to RAM and processor speeds? Do we need this trickle-down method of medicating the rich … as the poor gets treatment only decades later? We are SO marketed for "bigger is better" that nobody stops to question the numbers and the necessities of society before buying into something "bigger".

Innovations take inventions and make it available to the masses. It took years for normal people to afford quad-core phones with a 12.1-megapixel camera; whilst the rich are going out and buying phones with processors that are constantly "ground-breaking"; the flagships.

I know only a few people in the world, and less companies, who are thinking of sustainable solutions to flagship materialisms. If I am criticizing innovations that "fix" problems of societies, what more do I expect people to do to maintain and (hopefully) evolve society?

Most of the problems of the maintenance of society do not involve innovations. As mentioned earlier, innovation and invention are mostly for the advantages of the rich (or the few). Societal and mental problems, such as recycling and commercial wastes and access to education, are based mostly on post codes and zoning areas, which are controlled by the government and the illuminati types. This affects the health of the society as a whole, and are commonly ignored by the society of the few.

Deceitful press, negative marketing and political barriers are usually the mainstay of the stagnant situations people are in. I mentioned that statistics are hockey-sticking upward, but nations seem to have a snail's pace in evolving to take advantage of examples from other more advanced nations.

As I walk around Malaysia, I realize that the mentality and culture of the status quo seem to be adopting the worst of other nations. I hear people proud to say that "we have Five Guys now!" and "We have Taco Bell!" They seem to be proud to promote the fact that they have adopted the lowest side of societal ideals, and that is illogical to me.

I have even seen a Perodua Myvi converted to a Daihatsu. Because it is "better" to have a foreign-branded car instead of a local one. However, my headaches come from the fact that everyone knows it is a Myvi, and that Daihatsu is not the best of car brands. It is just marketed to the people that foreign materialisms MUST be better.

This is the type of mentality that keeps people from questioning the government, and stops people from realizing the governmental barriers that block the adoption of innovations that promote social, environmental and humanitarian justices. I have seen this type of behavior in almost every country I have been to and lived in.

However, in some countries, critical mass makes a difference. More advanced nations – not the outdated concept of "first-world" nor the racist concept of "Western nations" – who have more forward-thinking peoples, have been able to advance societal and mental health by transparently marketing physical, social and mental health concepts to their populations.

A critical mass is needed to create positive changes, adopt innovations that promote sustainability, and fight for equality and equity for all peoples. Society then is in the hands of the many, instead of in the hands of the few. That makes a positive 180° shift (a revolution is 360° shift in which nobody wins) from the stagnant societies we live in now.

Personally, I wish there were more people anticipating problems. In my hobby of people-watching, it seems that people are bouncing off bumpers until they ultimately fall into the trough. If people take the initiative to be socially active and interact with the "icky" people outside their social classes, then there would be more empathy.

Once there is understanding of peoples' problems and issues, there would be an initiative to fix physical, social and mental issues facing society; especially the societies that I have seen in developing countries, such as Malaysia, Croatia, et alia.

Culturally, Croatia and Malaysia and most Arabic League nations have something in common. That is not to share problems outside their own personal space. Other populations might also relate to this, but I am writing from my experiences. Talking about problems is still taboo. Going to a psychiatrist or psychologist could get you disowned or fired.

Mental changes are attributed to not being religious enough in these societies, and mental illnesses are attributed to being *possessed*. In the 21st century and in the times of scientific knowledge and understanding, I am more amazed by the 16th century mentality of ignorant persons who put outdated, theological beliefs over evidence-based, scientific theories.

A friend once said, "Yeop, not everybody is you!"

I wish they were, so there would be no need for me to write about social justice, and concentrate more on arcane alternative medicine in different regions of the world.

Heal the World

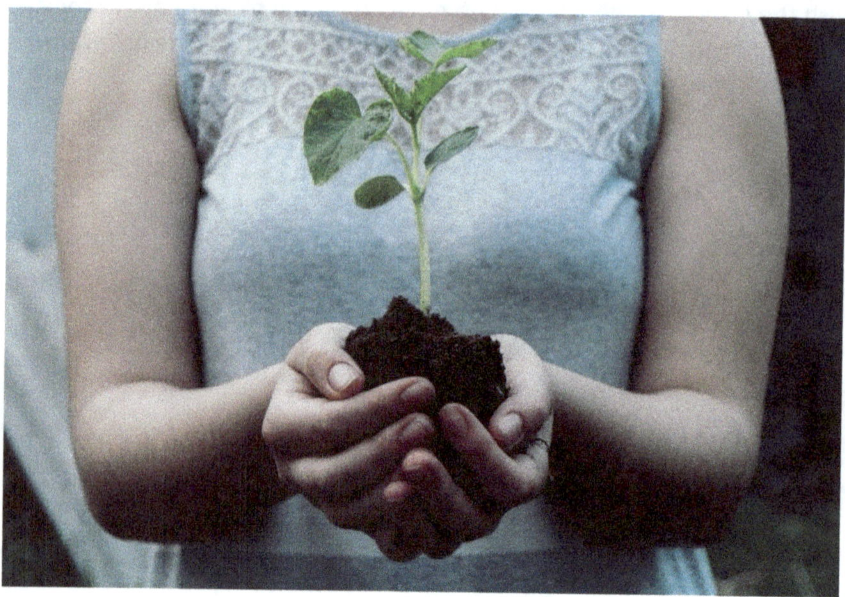

As I recovered in Malaysia and spoke to the locals, I realized people fall into three different "categories". We are all born equal, even for a split second, but are eventually nurtured into a box that fits our local societies. Only a few of us are able to break free. Either by having escaped the box at a young age (like me), or even deserving of more respect, having an imagination that is outside the box, and creating a path out of goals and dreams.

The **first** type of people, who exit the box, are usually the people involved in innovation. These are the dreamers, those who can create and evolve society in the right direction (thankfully, there were not a lot who evolved us in the wrong direction). Albeit, I met a few who struggle to get back into the box and try to bring others with them.

These people take initiative in manipulating their surroundings to fix problems, to lobby for solutions, and change laws for the better of nature and eventually humanity. There are many obstacles, and these people are usually quiet in the implementation of their ideas. A little step here, a lot of steps there.

The hardest part is to convince the critical mass, which move like molasses so that each step in a positive direction might take generations. Take banning of leaded fuel and lead paints as an example. Those policies took forever to implement, despite the proof to be a significant cause of IQ loss.

On the other hand, the initiative to eradicate smallpox was amazing; to create and implement policies to save the world from a pandemic. It was a miracle that people worked together (I am sure there were struggles). It was also amazing that they managed to organize house visits to 120 million households per month in India, and coordinated cooperation between USA and Russia at the height of the cold war!

More than 1/5th into the 21st century, the innovators that I got to know in the 1990s appear to be hindered by religious, political and economic limits. The brilliance of humanity seems to get less funding than those who market to the status quo. Instead of investing more of the GDP into inventors, innovators and long-term endeavors, most governments only see four (or five) years into the future of their countries.

Many governments see less into environmental issues, and concentrate more into materialistic goods such as real estate and housing developments, which is being built in a rate that is more than the needs of humanity.

These days, we can only name a handful of forward-thinking people. And sometimes, we mock them. Or we do not give them recognition. I hardly know anyone who followed the launch of the James Webb, let alone marvel at the first images, let alone know who James Webb is. People seem tethered to the ground, and are suddenly blind-sided by the repercussions of the status quo of their older generations.

The **second** type of people are involved in maintenance of the box. These are the blue-collar laborers. Most shifted from factory grounds into cubicles; from repetitive robotic labor to a form of repetitive number crunching. These people are at the most risk of being automated, but lobby for their careers with strong labor unions.

Despite the simplicity of their jobs, they act to maintain prestige by masking themselves in suits and briefcases. They sit in meetings with their laptops and tablets, and watch statistical graphs that are manipulated at their axes.

Their only job is to maintain the status quo, and make the critical mass feel comfortable. Instead of Utopian thinking, they keep drilling for oil, pumping gas, making plastics, create monocrop plantations, and then go home to their nuclear families to tell them about their nine-to-fives. A concept formed in the 1950s and has not evolved in over 70 years.

Real estate, number of cars, and brand names measure wealth for them, and there is a fierce – albeit hushed – competition between neighbors and families based on competitive jealousy. Capitalism, they wrongly call it. I have lived through this, and refused to join the game, and have ridden my bicycle nearly daily since I was 12 when I got my first bicycle. I also walk everywhere, which is shameful because I am then considered a commoner.

This group of people do not just maintain the critical mass, they ARE the critical mass, who need to be herded into the next innovative viewpoint. They, however, hold the power since they are the majority; and the majority wins elections. Governments, with their short-sighted plans, then must only maintain the happiness of the critical mass to enslave them within the mindset of the status quo.

In my travels, every citizen is boasting about their nation's infrastructure without realizing the impact of what the nation has just built. The Merdeka Tower, for instance, should have not been built. Skyscrapers are useless in today's environmental changes, and create more of a carbon footprint for the nation and its people.

However, the group of people, who work their nine-to-five to maintain status quo, hardly question outside their nuclear way of life. They create the market for the third type of people.

Finally, the **third** type of people are involved in promoting the box.

This is every business or political tactic, and this is how the world functions. Unfortunately, good people work haphazardly, and are less coordinated than established corporations. In the 21st century, the world is hockey-sticking itself towards better statistics, but what are we doing with those statistics?

Those hockey-stick statistics create contentment for the critical mass, and the Utopian views of the first types have again reached a brick wall.

There are many crises around the world, which are relatively isolated and unrelated (at least to us non-illuminati). Most people have more than enough. We have more than five camels worth, so we should be able to embrace a shifting world population with tolerance and understanding. Especially with the entire knowledge of the world at our fingertips!

However, the trend that I have seen in my world travels has been that nations have become more nationalistic, people have collapsed into selfishness, and the world has followed corporate thinking to market sweet frosting to the critical mass and divert from social problems. Underneath that frosting, the cake still tastes like *$h!t*.

A friend and mentor of mine once said that, "Grass will always be greener on the other side, the secret to life is to make your grass greener."

Classifying people into categories have historically created complicated "situations", and you cannot (and should not) put people into strict classifications. People fall into spectrums, and populations fall into a spectrum of all three.

I still drive a fossil fuel car for long distances, and I drive alone. Nobody is there with me to carpool. I still maintain other forms of environmental maintenance as nature provides for us all. I would love to get people to come with me, but these days, communication between people in communities is just slightly above asocial. Generations of humans seem lost as we cornered into the 21st century.

At this point of humanity (actually, we should have started changes in the 1970s), people must realize that the first step into becoming closer to being the first type of person is – with every movement, every decision, every action – to always question:

"How can I make this better?"

Metabolic Placebo

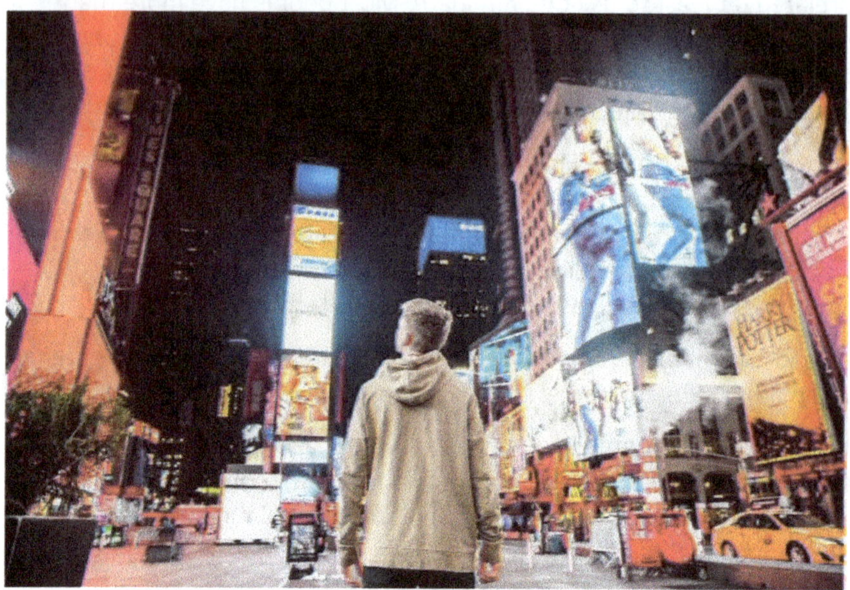

I wanted to write about the placebo effect, but my boss from work told me to write about a problem facing most modern societies; **the metabolic syndrome**. The metabolic syndrome encompasses the change in our metabolism due to external forces that is associated with atherosclerosis, heart disease, obesity, diabetes, inflammation, stroke, bone degradation and many other symptoms or diseases which are intertwined.

One can write individual chapters about each disease, and the solutions to tackle each problem, which is what most modern medicine does. One has high blood pressure; there is a pill (or combinations) for it. If you have type II diabetes, you take a pill (or combinations) for it. As you get closer to the end of your natural life, the pharmaceutical industry gets richer. I am not saying that pharmaceutical-based medications are bad, or that they do not work, but the metabolic syndrome is a multi-discipline topic that most hospitals and specialists address individually.

People have this stigma against general practitioners, because we seem to just refer patients to specialists for specialized examinations. However, we are the few primary care physicians who have to know almost everything, and find the common denominator that tie these diseases together. Unless someone has a rare, genetic predisposition to a disease (like Tetralogy of Fallot or certain cancers as an extreme example), there are simple solutions to live a long, pain-free and healthy life.

Unfortunately, bad advertising is stronger.

When I moved to Croatia, many people told me that they are who they are because they pick their own individual self. They make their own decisions, and so they are special. However, people forget about advertising influencing the decisions that steer their lives. Why then do the majority of Europeans smoke? Because their friends do? Is it peer pressure? It is no coincidence that children, despite evidence-based medicine and advertising proving smoking is directly linked to lung cancer, will start smoking because their parents are smokers. There is even an ad on cigarette packages advertising that claim.

Do we pay attention?

Unfortunately, not most of us.

Metabolic Placebo

So why not make my own term and call it **metabolic placebo**? There are many aspects of life that allow people to live healthy, and those things must be advertised and socially accepted. When a new diet comes out and are read in magazines, or it comes on their mobile news feed, most people will follow that trend, because it worked for the few people writing the article, or are getting monetized on YouTube. The keto-diet, intermittent fasting, Ramadan, etc.

The human body is not built that way. The human body is a machine. Metabolic syndrome causes different symptoms, but a single cell individually does not have many functions. However, they work together to create who you are: a series of neuronal connections that control a physical machine that is programmed to shove stuff into your face hole and discard what it cannot use out your butt hole. This action, advertised by multi-national industries, are major causes of metabolic syndromes in the western world, and it is considered a social-determinant of health in developing countries, such as in Croatia.

When people read these things, they choose to follow advertising, and it becomes a trend or a fad that they will do for a few months or years, before falling back to tradition and culture. Depending on the traditions and cultures of the region you live in, this could be a good change, or it could cause the basis of metabolic syndromes.

One example of a great anti-oxidant that reduces inflammation, aging and aging body pain associated with daily use of your "machinery", is turmeric. I got asked by lady in Croatia if they should buy these extremely expensive turmeric pills, because in India, people are less obese and statistically have less heart diseases compared to the western world.

I told them it works in India, because Indians eat curry for breakfast, lunch and dinner. I doubt that people here would change their lifestyle and diet to do that in Europe, nor in any other parts of the world where turmeric is not a daily staple; even though it would change their metabolism for the better, placebo or not. People follow fads, not lifestyle changes.

How do you treat metabolic syndrome? You can create and advertise good fads and trends. Even though people think that they are making their own choices, they subconsciously follow fads and trends. Unfortunately for most developed and faster-developing countries, fast-food and delivery is more convenient, multi-national companies have more money to advertise, and that Popeye's chicken sandwich is SO GOOD! Integrating apps to simply order processed foods makes things worse.

Recycling good fads and trends could then be the solution or placebos that make people believe they are living well.

Not too long ago (relatively), I would be considered unhealthy for being thin. Parents and grandparents would tell me that I should eat more, but I have kept the same figure and relative strength since high school. Sure, there are aging problems, and some parts that I used more wear down quicker, but my choice was made by the fact that I watched my peers get worse. I would talk about my problems, my pains, and as a scientist, I would like to see how my body gauges compared to others at my age.

I obviously cannot compare myself to YouTubers, who are there to advertise their fads, get fans and monetize their channel. However, I can compare myself to the critical mass of the country I live in, or the normal individuals I keep in touch with internationally.

The Placebo Effect

What is the placebo effect? In simplicity, the placebo effect is a psychosomatic cause when "things" influence your brain to create reactions in your body, either positive or negative (nocebo effect). Joe Scott gave a lot of interesting examples and explains what the brain can release by giving a placebo and making a person believe they are being medicated. An example in his video was a person went through knee surgery, where the surgeon did not do anything except for cutting it open, and suturing it back up. The knee apparently got better.

As Joe mentioned, people prefer a big machine more than surgery, which is then better than an injection. I have personal experiences in this. Injections works better than a capsule, and a pill works better than a doctor's explanation that generics are the same as branded products. Pill colors and physician confidence also makes a big difference. I personally have this problem, because I look young and few patients listen to me until they realize that I am forty and am a veteran doctor. Being clean-shaven also makes a big difference for some odd reason.

Although the placebo effect is mostly mentioned in medicine and research, there have been multiple studies done that placebo now almost have the same effect as the medications themselves. However, placebos can be anything. As mentioned before, the colors of pills can affect the human mind and make the body react differently. An interesting example was a woman with irritable bowel syndrome, who entered a study knowing she was taking a placebo. Through the study and taking the placebo, she had no symptoms. Then those symptoms came back after the trial ended.

Little do people know in Croatia, who know me only as a medical doctor, is that I graduated and worked as a biochemist. I worked in phase I clinical trials in North Carolina before deciding to advance my career in medicine. In this time, we tested the absorption of drugs in a double-blind study, where some people got placebos and some people got the real medication. I cannot really go into detail of what we did, but there have been many studies that have said that those medications were only slightly effective over the placebo.

Having our "subjects" stuck in a clinic over a weekend and conversing with each other might have had an effect on the symptoms of the drug tested. Some people might feel an effect, and the others listening to him or her might automatically feel the same effect or side-effects. Power of suggestion can create effects on people that other people subconsciously pick up.

Even in relationships, a guy can be a solid 6 or a solid 7, and just having a good wing man, you immediately look and feel like an 8 or even end up a perfect guy for a girl you would never meet on your own.

Suggestion and advertising are powerful, and "we are often judged by the company we keep".

There are a few key hormones and neurotransmitters released in the body, which effect the body in either positive or negative ways. Some people do feel awful after smoking a cigarette after reading that "Smoking Kills" or having pictures of anatomical body parts they do not recognize.

Do they want to have that? No.

Some people will smoke less and eventually (and hopefully) stop, despite my previous statement, there are less smokers. Africa had problems against tobacco lobbyists when trying to do the same advertising to lessen the smoking population.

Advertising Healthcare

Does it work? This is the reason that the field of **public health** exists. These doctors are also the hidden heroes, who can save millions by *advertising*. Unfortunately, doctors are not as creative as multi-national companies, that spend millions of monies that most social governments or Ministries of Health do not have, to empower, lobby or educate the masses on national or global level.

Do we have to advertise a common-sense lifestyle that can reverse a simple problem like metabolic syndrome?

Do we have to tell someone to stop smoking and advertise the reasons to do so?

Do we have to tell them that they are too fat, and that they must care about their risk of diabetes, cardiovascular diseases, and stroke?

Did the food pyramid have an effect (which was wrongly placed with processed carbohydrates being on the second level) on people eating fast and processed foods?

Are all foods now processed even though they are home-cooked?

Most foods these days are GMOs, despite (through news and advertising) people being aware of avoiding GMOs. Cooking anything at home is the same as processing raw foods and will change protein structure, but somehow it works well for people to believe that it does not.

Is this the metabolic placebo that people tend to believe in? For most of the people, does it create a healthy lifestyle to prepare a home-cooked meal? How do health-aficionados think individual proteins are extracted, and then re-added as an "additive" to their apparently healthy shakes they take in the mornings?

Most everybody is looking to live a better and longer life in fear of death. Since I work in emergency medicine, death seems very taboo to people despite most people being religious, and realizing that death is inevitably a part of life. If people die of natural causes such as the case of metabolic syndrome, the blame goes on the physician or caretaker, and people will try to blame doctors or caretakers as much as possible to psychologically create a scapegoat. People tend to forget, as Bill Burr mentioned in one of his stand-ups, that he was not the one shoving burgers into their face-holes for years.

Despite the society's lack of knowledge and the declining respect of doctors, extending the average lifespan from around 50 years old in the 19th century to close to 90 years old in 2020, people must realize that doctors and science do make a difference, but cannot be there with the person 100% of the time to constantly tell them that the things they do are not optimally healthy.

It would be like an engineer driving your car for you, and fixing each tiny problem as they come along. When was the last time you checked your brakes? Do you pay attention when your belts start squealing? When you take it to the mechanic, and your engine timing is off due to your own ignorance, do you blame the mechanic for a shorter engine life or even a car crash?

You must empower yourself and create a better lifestyle, or suffer the fate of disease and early death. As with a car, your body will age and it will wear down. The only difference is that your body can sometimes fix itself, and it is a just a bio-machine for your brain.

By comparing your body at 42 with your body at 36, when most metabolic processes start to change, you will notice differences and will start taking pills to lower blood pressure, reduce risk of stroke and treat the symptoms of diabetes, but most people do not take care of themselves as much as they take care of their car.

Which is OK.

You can still feel healthy. By reducing stresses of life, and living in a normal human society, your brain can and will release hormones, endogenous chemicals, and neurotransmitters (endorphins, dopamine, serotonin, and histamines) that reduce both pain and help with metabolic syndrome; as long as, you take care of yourself like you take care of your car. Change your liquids regularly, check your levels, and things will work for a long time.

In my years of work, I have seen fat people with no diabetes live until an old age, and I have seen skinny people, who force themselves daily, die early with a heart attack. Placebo works only a little less than real medication, and older medications worked better than placebo. To have the placebo effect of better health, **quality of life** can be affected by mental advertising, personal psychological responses to environment, reduction of stress, and better powers of suggestion.

Does it Work? Really?

Why not try Yoga or Tai Chi for a start? Meditation and power of thought is a very powerful thing. Obviously, placebos cannot only solve problems such as cancer and fight certain infections, but it can lower symptoms and increase immunity. Placebo is neurologically and psychosomatically tricky, because your environment and exposure to senses can be influenced so easily. In a simple experiment, you can change your own conscious experiences.

Try making things "brighter" just by opening your eyes wider, letting more natural light in. If you feel sad, go out into the sun, and notice those colors that you are attracted to. Wear those colors that you enjoy. Take a long shower and make yourself pretty. Endorphins will get released, and you will feel better about yourself. It will not solve deeper depression, but it does change moods, and your overall condition, and maybe immunity, would improve through these psychosomatic effects.

When I have things to do and go for a walk or run my errands, I honestly do not feel my shoulder pain. Belief, goals and social interactions can reduce pain. It is not just "ignoring" pain, but due to the release of endogenous hormones and natural opioids during social interactions, your pain will subside. It also happens when you fall in love, and dopamine is released. It may create a sensation of invincibility, and that pain you have felt for years can go away. Especially in those first few "loving" months.

I sometimes tell my patients that they just need love.

Confidence in medicine, the way doctors present themselves as authoritative figures – as mentioned earlier – usually work better even before medication is given. Laughter, according to Dr. Patch Adams (yes, he is real), has shown to decrease symptoms for cancer patients, who experience constant pain. What he does is to utilize natural antidepressants, pain relief, naturally increase metabolic processes in the body, etc.

In my experience, the most important medication to patients is acknowledgement and empathy. That is why good psychologists should be more integrated into society, despite the taboo of seeing a psychiatrist or psychologist in religious and developing countries.

In the 1980s and 1990s before smartphones, apps and the need for "quick acknowledgement" through "likes", people had time for each other and sharing problems and stories were free psychotherapy. Everyday things were slower, and daily social acknowledgement was the placebo that could lower the use of anti-depressants.

Depressed people usually are stagnant and are at high risk for metabolic syndromes. Now people are in a rush to get absolutely nowhere. Then they work overtime for a paycheck to buy materialistic things that makes them feel better by temporarily increasing endorphins instead of taking the time to socialize.

Metabolic Syndrome Through Placebo

Acknowledgement, love, a simple life, social support, friendly competition, tolerance, acceptance, and taking the time to empathize with people would bring back people to the older days before today's screen-based technology.

Who should be responsible for all this?

Family doctors, general practitioners and public health have more contact with patients, and can empower people to have confidence in themselves, exercise regularly, teach them to eat healthier to decrease the risk of metabolic syndromes.

I just read that *WORLDWIDE*, society is missing 4.3 million physicians, most of them being primary care physicians. It is up to lay persons to "believe" that our poorly advertised public service announcements will work. I see people buy turmeric pills, drink their kale shakes, intermittent fast, drink a ton of water, and feel better despite not finding any concrete evidence-based medicine on the topics.

Despite being fat, having a weak heart, having high blood pressure, etc., people can believe that this is their cultural norm, reduce their stress level, and maybe the placebo effect will make a difference in the **quality of life**, which is what we should be aiming for.

"Loneliness is often the product of a gifted mind."

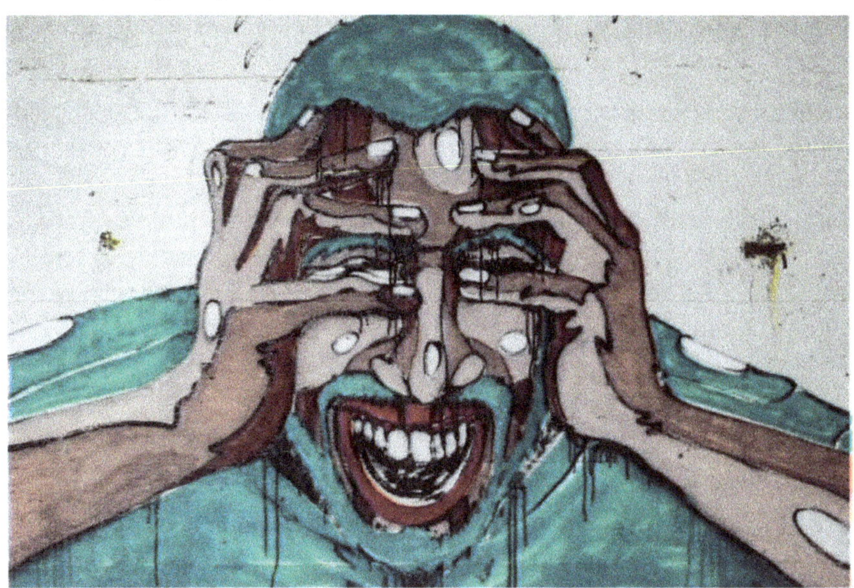

I will probably be mislabeled as egotistical and pushing my own agenda towards my own means of survival. However, this society has clearly misunderstood many people with intelligence willing to push for changes that they see wrong in their surroundings. They are suppressed and categorized into labels, so they can be further medicated to fit into today's society.

It is hard to understand the minds and thought processes of people who can think at a million miles a minute. Even though I feel my mind is fast, there are many minds that are faster, and I too fear them. Not because I fear what they can do. I fear that I cannot keep up.

The only way that I can absorb them is to slow down the wonders that they present. Take them one at a time and let my own brain organized them. It is lucky that most of these people have good intentions. There are people who explore space, create new ways to sustain this planet, and put their own efforts above their own desire to just survive.

While they create wonders, the majority of the people forget that these people are still human. They still make mistakes, but they learn from them and use those opportunities to rectify. They do things to bring themselves to society – to seem almost human – so that they are not considered outcasts within their surroundings.

Should they suppress themselves, so that they are understood? Or should society take the time to pick up their "smart" phones, do a little research, and understand them? There are only a few of them, who take the time to bridge the gap. Personally, I read and watch the videos to understand the marvels that they create. Those marvels, which allow people to scroll through memes, get stuck and complain about the traffic that they themselves cause, or the overabundance of nutrition they put on their own plates and eventually throw into the trash. Unseparated.

These problems that societies themselves cause create newer problems, which people of intelligence must deal with. There are only a few of them who question those problems. Most people flush their toilets without marvel of where their own excrements go. What if you have an entire village flushing their excrements into the system? What if you have an entire megapolis flushing their toilets?

It is very detrimental to the environment to release that much waste into rivers and oceans, most not caring what happens downstream from them. Most do not care what happens to lower society living in the filth of the upper class. There are only a few of them who create solutions, but they are usually ignored, mocked and cast aside. Only a few survive and create something, through clever marketing, to make the people – who are blindly stuck in the rat race – switch over.

Peoples do not like to break out of their comfort-zone. They gladly climb within their level by buying the "biggest" and the "best" of what their society is bounded by. They do not like to think of the downstream. Why think about what could happen in 2030, when they enjoy their "now"?

What is admirable is that some of these game-changers do not even have children to bring into the new generation. They fight for changes to bring salvation to humanity's children. They will fight for the bigger picture; while societies slowly benefit from their work; usually not realizing that most of these miraculously modern efforts put affordable food on the table, roofs above their heads, clean water from their pipes, and clothes on their backs.

People fear change, even if it is for the better. I see this in every society that I have had the privilege to live in. From being stuck in traffic, because people decide to not follow the rules; to losing life and love, because people are tied down to their narrow band of societal pressures. These days, it takes more than just a thought to get out of the box. It takes a step and a fight against societal norms. People have become too comfortable in their hedonism to take that leap, and need a metaphorical slap in the face to do so.

However, there is no more need for preaching and lectures.

I am one of many repeating the message from the same broken record. It is time for people to decide to think about the others and to work together as a society, instead of embracing the fact that they are merely controlled by a paycheck and the fear of loss of it. So strong is that fear, they do not take a step towards better gains. Towards knowledge. Too many times have we been manipulated and hypnotized by our 5" brains in the palm or our hands, that we absorb even the worst without any fact checks.

I was nurtured as a scientist, and that comes with a curse of cynicism to any fact that comes across my senses. I am the type to never say no until it has been tried. I would fact check even my own birth. I have caused anger and resentment among people by undermining their beliefs with facts; much to the point where I have been treated as a nothing. My own family is ashamed to talk about me, because despite my accomplishments, I have broken their belief structure. I stepped outside their system. I am not even hated; that requires acknowledgement. To them, I am a nothing.

That is today's society. Living in bliss of the ignorance of the faults that they themselves cause. Climate changes, systemic racism, social inequalities, etc. Most people I know live without consequence to themselves, and they ignore the consequences to the bottom rung of the social ladder. People are marketed to live in the *NOW!* and the *FUTURE!*, but people seem to forget to learn from their past; as these problems are shoved back down until they reemerge stronger and louder than before.

The few have created wonders for the norms to exploit. These norms then trickle down their wealth to those who fear loss. Then they trickle down further, until there is nothing left at the bottom. Hardly anything makes it to the people who have lost and/or have to start with nothing.

We, the nothing, do not fear loss, as we have nothing to lose except for our lives. And for a few, not even that. I have lost half my life to the whim of those who enforce, those who promote societal norms, those who hold pride for false ideals. I have lost to people who hold higher positions on the social ladder, to social 'normalities' of skin pigmentation, and I have lost a lot in compensating for others who do not even care about the planet they live on.

Yet, I can live a life of high moral grounds, despite my immoral doings to get to that height. I had to lie, steal and cheat the system to, in a bigger picture, display truths, distribute wealth, and fight for equity and equality. For the people of the lower rung. In my mind, when I step back, I see the fault in the advertising and marketing to these 'normals'. The power, held by corporations who control their choices, is constantly abused. I feel sad when I see people choose wrongly instead of wisely. For it does not take much, these days, to choose wisely.

"Why should I step down, when I could step up?"

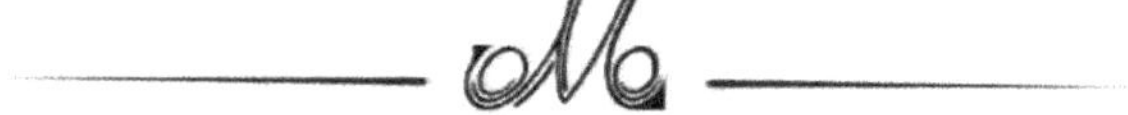

A Personal Example

This aggravates me, and gives me a headache.

The Malaysian government is known not to have signed the 1951 Refugee Convention nor its 1967 Protocol and does not have a legislative or administrative framework to protect refugees and asylum seekers within its jurisdiction. This means that most of the support comes from NGOs, mainly UNHCR and private donors who give the minimal support. Refugees are not allowed to work nor are they allowed to register nor are they allocated healthcare and education. The government is keen on kicking them out, and will as soon as they are caught with minimal cause.

I have been there. Not having anything. Being a nothing.

I talked about not paying Zakat (alms) to the Zakat committee, because they are usually corrupt. Any organizational money collector has some corruption. I rather know where my money goes, and do individual payments in the name of alms and donations. My mother then says that they do not need support, because they are the ones who break into houses. They are not welcome here. Why should they come to Malaysia?

This gave me a headache when I had to listen to this in Europe. People were fleeing war zones, persecution and poverty. They needed to make a better life for their future generations, and not just themselves. This seemed to be lost in the minds of the upper classes; upper from where I am.

I had to walk out of there, because I felt anger swell up. I told her that this is not a conversation to be had. It is one thing to live in ignorance of the misfortunate; it is another thing to promote the abandonment of them.

Environmental Health

Earth Day Star-date NOW!

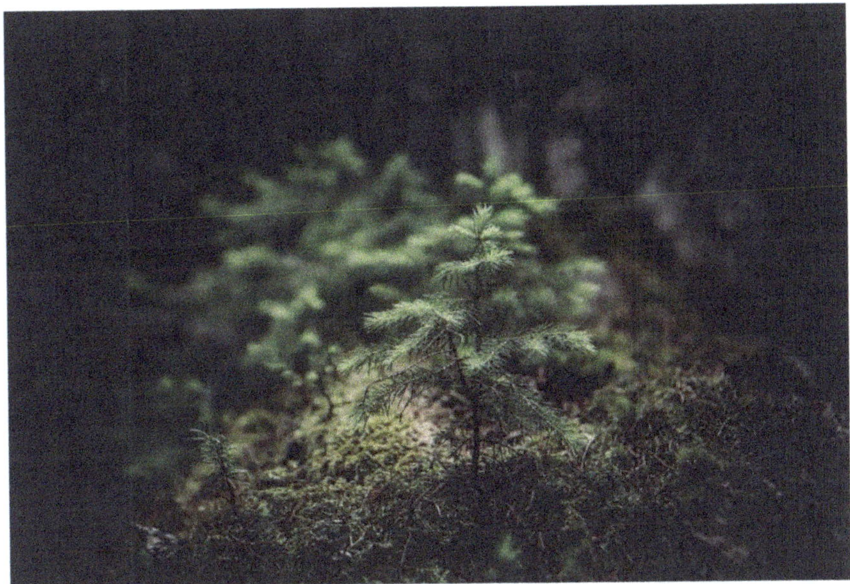

Earth day is one of those arbitrarily designated days, much like Valentine's Day, that should not be a celebrated day if everybody had common sense. Taking care of the environment should be habit. Dying are the days of Henry Ford and Thomas Midgley, Jr. when gasoline had become king. Even in the 1980s and 1990s, people were more environmentally conscious, and I remember taking our garbage to the recycling center with our neighbors to recycle as much as we can.

Yes, Europe. In America, the neighbors got together, filled up a truck with recyclables and drove it to the recycling center. We took turns. It was more social.

The World Health Organization defines health, not only in the absence of disease, but in the promotion of physical, mental, social ... plus **environmental** and spiritual health. All these aspects of health must be in balance for a person to live a higher quality of life, which is the goal of many societies. Although I could delve into the atrocities of today's physical, mental, social (*gawk!*) ... and spiritual, you will probably be asking, "Why is the environment important for good health?"

This is a big task to unravel, and – like any complicated issue – is multi-factorial. Environmental health ranges from public health measures (i.e., clean water, sewage treatment, etc.); to real estate zoning to reduce social injustices (racism); to promoting equity and equality for ALL people to get access to human necessities. These are things we do not think about; at least most of us.

The poor think that they have no other options; the rich do not think about the living conditions of the poor. This is not only a problem for the poor, but the wealthy have expanded their real estate into the natural habitats of even aborigines (*orang asli*) and dislocating them from their heritage and lands.

How is this related to a pandemic? Most viruses are zoonotic in nature. Viruses can mutate at an amazing speed and due to errors in their copying process, they can evolve into a strain that can jump to other species, and spread their infection type further. This was true of SARS-CoV-2 and it will be true again; probably in the near future.

These human habits of destroying nature, mono-cropping, deforestation for grazing, plastic pollution, climate change, and many other abominations to the planet that peoples have done over the past 200 years, have not helped our health as a society at all. This has not only extinguished key species, but also had left many animal species homeless.

However, we can prevent and eventually (hopefully) reverse this by realizing that deforestation leads to displacement of animals, but life goes on. Nature is intelligent enough to work with changes, change their genetics, and move from natural jungles to concrete ones (the jungle where humans live); many of which carry viruses ready to make that zoonotic link.

There are MANY simple solutions that the critical mass of people can start doing THIS very second. It just takes a decision to do it. Most people just have to stop and think, "How can I do this better? **How can I MAKE this better?**" and pick the choice that is beneficial to others and not just themselves. Many countries and cultures are not as forward thinking when it comes to the environment. For example, people are still stuck on diesel engines. Let us praise the people who are leaping to zero(-ish)-emission electric vehicles.

In most countries – culturally – having many cars (and bigger engines) is a sign of wealth and status. More advanced nations, however, have realized that wealth has nothing to do with outward appearances. Understanding and knowledge begets wealth and status, but I have heard many people mock world leaders when they do proper things that are considered poor or common. I also have this problem when I walk in Malaysia.

How do we change?

Make a conscious decision.

From today, we can just **walk** to the store instead of drive. From today, we can ride our **bicycles** the next time we need to run a quick errand. From today, we can start to slowly switch to **public transportation** to get to work.

We can drive less to reduce carbon emissions. Easily enough, this also promotes that healthy lifestyle, which people spend hundreds of monies to go to the gym for. Most people I know even drive there, because they cannot fathom to get to the gym sweaty. It is easy to make these switches, but the human brain finds excuses not to. There are no more tomorrows. We have made that excuse too many times.

In my experiences, "**There is never a next time**."

Personally, I have made a rule that if the total is 5 kilometers (3.2 miles), I will walk it. If the total is about 12 kilometers, I will bike it. If it is anything over 12 kilometers, then I can use my car (I wish I had a motorbike). I also only use my car to get to work (100 km away with no public transportation), and when I go grocery shopping once every two weeks. Many people can make these rules, and I would be proud of you if your distances are better than mine.

Home gardening, and being around plants and nature have been linked to decreased stress levels. A gardening experience promotes a sense of purpose and repetition, which forms habit in a healthy way. It is important for peoples to return to a more natural lifestyle, as an alarming number of kids seem to think that milk comes from the fridge.

An adult should also focus on eating less ranch-grazed meats and concentrate on vegetables, which are not monocrops. These corporate activities cause more deforestation than necessary. By avoiding monocrops and limiting meat, the society will be headed in the right direction to live healthier and more complete lives.

Realizing that nature is not there for abuse, and that humans are not viruses that destroy nature instead of symbiotically and harmoniously living among it, humanity can feel a sense of completion with their surroundings. This concept reduces stress and is the placebo needed to reduce metabolic syndromes. Nature, and especially trees, is known to reduce stress levels in people, therefore there is an importance for not only replanting trees, but also for forest preservation. Newer trees need at least 25 years to mature, and in that time, trees will release more carbon dioxide than use it, a fact that very few people know. The foliage of older trees and ancient forests are more important; thus, forest preservation is key while the lungs of the planet are being re-grown.

Science > politics. Always.

Good health is undoubtedly directly affected by the environment. Whether it be at the level of working as a community to maintain a social garden, or to replanting millions of trees to re-establish the carbon capture capacity of the planet, people must realize that there are many things needed to be done as daily chores to help our planet recover from centuries of abuse.

To create a sustainable future, common goals must easily be listed out (this has been done thousands of times before), so that people do not forget to do these tasks in each household. Within social aspect of mental health, we can all become a community again; open up and share problems. We need to practice tolerance and spirituality, because we are not the product of our nations, we are a product of a global whole.

In the 21st century, we are starting to realize that one corporation on one side of the world can affect the lives and livelihood of people on the other side, despite physical and social borders. Being in Malaysia (and most other countries I have lived in), there is an asocial aspect of life, which people need to change. Almost all religions promote goodness, so all peoples should practice acceptance and care. Especially towards nature, which will outlast us all.

Things people can easily do without excuses:

1. Sort the trash and recycle.

2. Start a food garden with your neighbors.

3. Clean your streets and neighborhoods - *no; the world is not your trash can, and it is not the government's responsibility to pick up your mess.*

4. Donate to re-plant trees.

5. Volunteer 2 hours a week to the refugees, homeless or even to clean up your neighborhood.

6. Think about what you eat, check for sustainability - *easy with smartphones.*

7. Think about what you buy, check for ethical sourcing - *easy with smartphones.*

8. Think if you really need to drive before you put your key in the door of your car.

9. Use a bicycle and slow down. Do not be in a rush to do absolutely nothing.

10. Breathe.

This is The Rhythm of The Night...

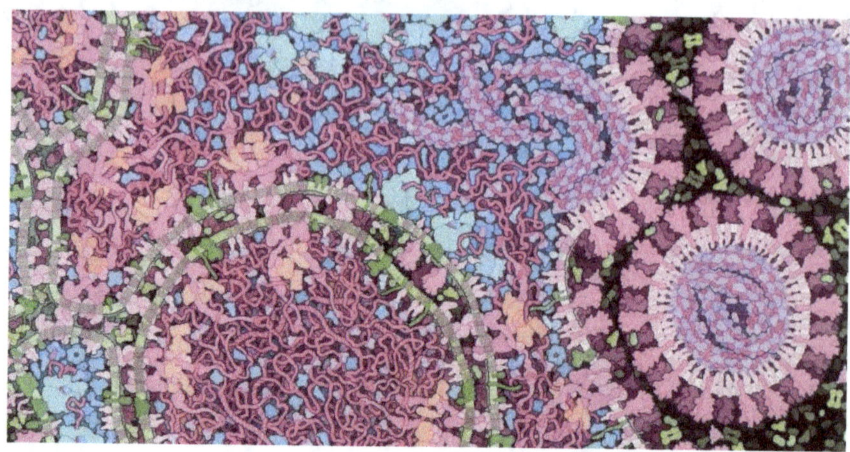

Illustrated by David S. Goodsell

After three years of the SARS pandemic, I am sure that nobody needs to know what COVID-19 is. However, a lot of people use it as a misnomer to what is spreading. COVID-19 is the sickness caused by the virus, SARS-CoV-2, which is one of many coronaviruses. Viruses. Viri?

Why is a pandemic an environmental issue? People quickly forget (*the past*) that zoonotic jumps in viruses and bacteria are usually due to changing the natural habitat of animals, forcing the more resilient creatures to migrate to the cities. *Yersinia pestis*, or the bubonic plague that killed **half of the world population** was due to an overabundant rat population due to the creation of cities

The lack of cleanliness in cities and pollution have also led to other outbreaks, such as cholera and dengue, which is still a common problem in the 21st century. We have not learned from the past, because we are too busy living in the present to think of the future

The pandemic is caused by a coronavirus, which is one of the most transmutable viruses. This means, it constantly changes its genetic makeup to create new types of infections almost every time it jumps from one host to another. It is believed that this virus is zoonotic, so there is no need for conspiracies against the Chinese government.

It happens.

Just like Ebola happens, HIV happens (which by the way is the world's largest and longest pandemic), and the yearly Influenza (flu) happens. Viruses mutate and they reinfect. How does this happen? They replicate so fast that at least one mistake in copying is made. Sometimes it is harmless; sometimes it causes another strain.

It is God's gamble with humanity.

This virus is designated SARS-CoV-2. S.A.R.S. actually stands for something. It is severe acute respiratory syndrome. It means that it primarily effects the lungs much like SARS-CoV-1. CoV stands for coronavirus, which is named after the spiky proteins on the outer coating of the virus. Corona means crown. Virus is a controversial "living" thing.

From the start, the World Health Organization did not want to ensue panic and economic failure across nations. It was not a slow response, and pandemic protocols have been written and revised since the Bush administration. However, this tactic did not work as people criticized the WHO, due to its cautious approach, to be in collaboration with China to spread the "man-made" virus all over the world. This tactic is known as finger-pointing, mostly amplified by a certain, fake-tanned, ex-president. I will not mention his name, because of his propensity to lawsuits.

The virus did not jump countries magically. This spread is due to close contact within circulated-air areas, such as buses, trains, planes and other forms of public transportation. It spreads much like the flu, where one person sneezes into the air and particulates will then spread and recirculate through AC units or fans, which are widely available in public transport. It just takes one person NOT to cover their nose and mouths for the virus to have a chance to get into the air instead of just your hand.

SARS-CoV-2 is quick like most flu viruses. It has a mean incubation period of 3 to 5 days. This means that, although the virus has already infected you and is starting to replicate, the symptoms will show up 3 to 5 days later, in which you could have already infected a few people. Therefore, masks work. And sometimes, it does not.

There are many types of masks out there, and obviously nobody is going to go around with their own oxygen supply and a HEPA filter attached to their face. Most people however are not taught how masks work, and how to wear a mask. The most common mask recommended is the N95 surgical masks. They stop 95% of particles that come out of your mouth. That is the point. They stop particles coming out of your mouth, when people wear them as they are. As a surgeon once told me, "Green always touches green."

Most people are not in the scientific field, but this is a pretty easy concept to grasp. The green end goes towards sterile, meaning that if you are sick, the green side goes towards the outside. If you are healthy and COVID-19 free, then the green side goes towards your face. This is because the masks are designed with one-way folds that catch particles. The way that most people wear masks is not effective, thus – despite wearing masks – the numbers of infections are still going up.

In addition to wearing masks, social distancing is a very effective way to slow down or stop the spread of any air-borne virus. The N95 masks will only slow down coughs or sneezes, so that most particles can only travel 30 centimeters. The recommended distance is two meters or six feet from the other person. However, in Asia, the distance is cut down to half that. It was pretty awkward for me to stand in lines at a distance of only one meter.

Why do I need a mask indoors?

Another good behavior to prevent any type of disease – not just COVID-19 – is to wash your hands regularly. This is the same message that we say for E. coli, cholera, and many other diseases. This works because of the structure of soap. Soap molecules are like little knives that cut through a membrane and break it apart. With agitation, it is like slashing multiple little knives into the capsules that surround a virus or bacterial membranes, leaving you with 0.1% bacteria or virus that is usually harmless. That is why hand-washing techniques are very important to follow, and the duration of hand-washing is important.

The rate of infection is referred to as the R-value, which is easy to understand. If one person can only infect another person, the R-value is 1:1 or 1. If they can infect two people, then the R-value is 2. This is very high, because the virus can quickly go from 1 to 2 to 4 to 8 to 16. This is clearly an exponential growth and that is why the population is not headed to recovery if the R-value is anywhere over 1. When the R-value is less than 1, then the virus is not being spread; thanks to interventions such as immunity from already been infected, isolation of the population (this is temporary and will only slow the R-value), and vaccines (this is more permanent).

Looking at the spikes of infections over time, there is a clear trend that follows most air-borne type viruses, such as influenza. There is a peak before the summer and a peak before the winter. These correlate to the times when people get together again, which can be easily avoided. This could be due to religious ceremonies, seasonal work, and especially schools. There is a very high correlation to the times when air-borne viruses hit and children going back to school.

Since children and the younger population are usually asymptomatic, they will lax on their usage of social distancing and masks, congregate in a classroom with others who might carry the virus, then bring them home to their individual households. Add to that a good 3 to 5-day incubation period, and the amount of contact that people have with other people. That will increase the chances of an exponential spread of any virus, not just SARS-CoV-2.

Anybody can get the virus, but the reactions of most people are asymptomatic (about 50%). However, there are risk factors that could increase the chances of hospitalization. In general, anything that causes chronic inflammation in your body could take away the body's ability to fight a new infection. In a sense, these additional infections could be labeled as a superinfection, making anybody with those risk factors worse.

Chronic inflammation is a wide definition. It could mean anything from cancer to diabetes to smoking. As long as someone has a risk factor, it is best to keep distances from anybody carrying a respiratory virus. This is a good general rule, not just for SARS-CoV-2. When someone else is sick, it is better not to be close to them.

There are long-term effects of the virus that are still being recorded, the most famous one being loss of smell and/or taste – anosmia. This is due to the virus being able to attack the upper respiratory tract, believed to be due to most people wearing masks BELOW the nose instead of fully covering their nose and mouth. There is a correlation between improper mask use and these upper respiratory tract symptoms. The other possible cause could be the return of virus to the upper respiratory tract by sneezing. Other long-term symptoms, to me, seem like psychological trauma.

Symptoms may develop 2 days to 2 weeks after exposure to the virus. A pooled analysis of 181 confirmed cases of COVID-19 outside Wuhan, China, found the mean incubation period was 5.1 days, and that 97.5% of individuals who developed symptoms did so within 11.5 days of infection.

The following symptoms may indicate COVID-19:

1. *Fever or chills*
2. *Cough*
3. *Shortness of breath or difficulty breathing*
4. *Fatigue*
5. *Muscle or body aches*
6. *Headache*
7. *New loss of taste or smell*
8. *Sore throat*
9. *Congestion or runny nose*
10. *Nausea or vomiting*
11. *Diarrhea*

Other reported symptoms include the following:

1. *Sputum production*
2. *Malaise*
3. *Respiratory distress*
4. *Neurologic (e.g., headache, altered mentality)*

Being unprepared for this type of acute respiratory syndrome, researchers and doctors and the entire medical field first had to figure out what the symptoms really were, and what the treatment is to reduce symptoms and stabilize the patient. That is why the WHO came up with "flattening the curve". Due to high rate of infection, the hospitals can be overrun by patients, and there are very limited breathing devices, medication, ICU beds, etc. Most everybody will get infected, but the most important thing is not to overwhelm the capacity of the system. That way, everybody can be treated. That is why it was important, in the early stages of the pandemic, to isolate.

As treatment goes, like most respiratory viruses, it is mainly supportive. The body will handle the virus on its own. There are antivirals that have been tried, corticosteroids to reduce over-inflammation responses (cytokine storm), and a lot of oxygen to get the body oxygenated. There are also physical treatments like putting the person in a reverse prone position to let the liquid in the lungs flow to the top of the lungs, so the bottom of the lungs (which has more surface area) can get some oxygen.

Other than that, doctors just maintain vitals (respiratory rate, heart rate, blood pressure, blood oxygenation, body temperature) and function of vital organs (brain, heart, lungs, liver, kidney, GI tract and spleen). Once your body is able to recover (or not), you're transferred into a normal ward (assuming you were in the ICU) for observation and further recovery. Low risk patients go home to isolation.

The vaccines are an amazing shift in modern medicine using mRNA, although the technology to target proteins in that way is pretty old. I remember people researching it when I was doing my Biochemistry degree. There is a video explaining what they have done and how it is amazing, and it can pave the way to creating vaccines for almost anything with knowledge of the target's DNA sequence. That is why this technology has not been used until now. It can be abused in a devastating way. People thought CRISPR was scary, but this can be even scarier.

What is mRNA vaccine?

Knowing the target protein of SARS-CoV-2, vaccines can be made to emulate those spike proteins (the ones creating the crown) → complicated biochemistry → and start an immune response in the body towards the encapsulated virus. This will not stop you from getting infected nor stop you from being viral, but it will not give you serious symptoms that will land you in the ICU.

That is why masks and social distancing is still needed, because many conspiracy theorists will not get vaccinated. The vaccines work in similar ways, but the best combination so far was found to be AstraZenica or Pfizer + Moderna or Novavax.

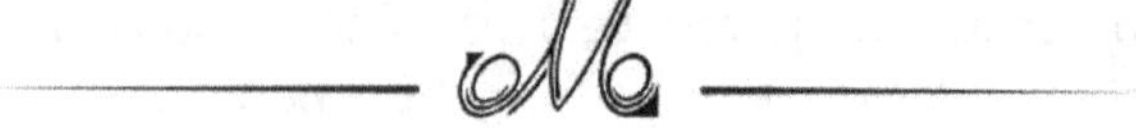

Currently, there are strains that are more infectious, but that does not mean more potent. The SARS part of the pandemic is slowing down, as the Omicron variant does not produce much SARS. The most important thing for people to do is to just wear masks and social distance indoors. There has been no correlation between masking outdoors and spreading the virus, unless you sneeze in that person's face. In that case, you would need to learn culture and manners. With cooperation, vaccination and QoL (quality of life) in consideration, governments and people will get through this pandemic better than the previous pandemics and epidemics.

Personally, I find it amazing that people have forgotten the other epidemics we have been through since the turn of the 21st century. Most people cannot name most of them. It is not the first time, nor will it be the last time. Learn from the past, do not live day by day, and prepare for the future, because that is best for your society and humanity as a whole.

Alternative medicine is always preventive medicine. There is no quick fix to sicknesses and diseases using alternative medicine. Alternative medicines do not even stop pain immediately. That said, any alternative medicine to combat SARS-CoV-2 involves boosting immunity, social distancing and making sure every individual is responsible enough to stop the spread of a contagious virus.

If zombies came at you, you would not want to get bitten. If you are infected, you do not want to go around biting people. Well, your brain would be mush, so you probably would.

Wear a mask, socially distance yourself, eat a healthy dose of Vitamin B, D and E (Vitamin C does not increase immunity), and think socially and responsibly to help humanity **flatten the curve** so that people who need the ICU get the ICU.

Disclosure

Good health can't just come from the ideas in this book. Those ideas are there as some alternatives that only require **small changes** in behavior for (hopefully) **big results**.

Each culture is different, and many parallels are available. On top of food and exercise and social understanding, health also requires simple prevention methods that is usually promoted by nine out of ten physicians.

Wash your hands.

Eat your vegetables.

Brush your teeth.

Wear a hat.

Epilogue

A Reminder for Doctors

We took an oath. For a long time, we forget that we are here to help and serve. We face high risk situations every day (especially working in rural Emergency Medicine), and even though we deal with hard problems daily, each day is no different than any other day we face. We are **soldiers** who have to answer the call.

Preventive medicine is promoted and advertised by the doctors in Public Health sectors. This will not change the prevalence of disease, but it gives researchers and healthcare professionals time to deal with each issue and not overwhelm the current healthcare infrastructure. Either way, deaths are inevitable. Medicine just delays death to a later time.

Until then, we need to **flatten the curve** of any disease to give the real heroes time to treat (*medical doctors and nurses*) or hopefully find a cure (*biochemists and researchers*).

After all, doctors are only the bartenders serving the *beer* that biochemists create.

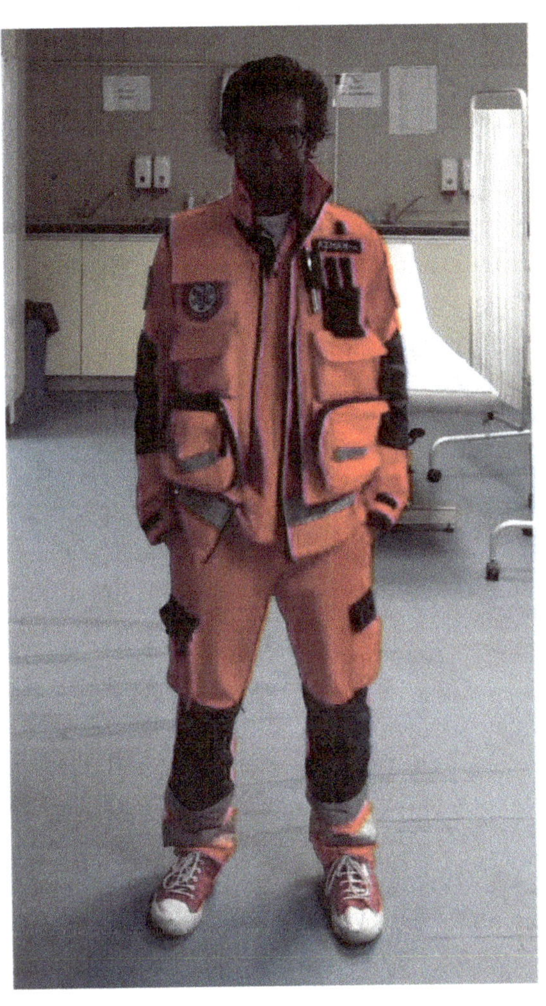

About the Author

My name is Yeop Azman. I would like to thank you for buying my first book! I was born on Wednesday, October 17, 1979 in the University Hospital in Kuala Lumpur. Because of my diplomatic parents, I have been to different places and cultures. From my birth in Malaysia, we have moved to and lived in Switzerland, the United States, Russia, and Germany.

I attended high school in Bonn, Germany at Bonn American High School, a Department of Defense Dependent School. I was there for the first three years of high school and was part of numerous activities, which I still do, and which define me as the person I am today. I then attended the International School of Kuala Lumpur for my senior year and graduated with two honors (NHS and Tri-M Music Honors) and 12 varsity letters in numerous sports and activities.

After graduation, I received a full scholarship from the Malaysian Government Public Service Department (JPA) to study pre-medicine abroad and with the "motivation" of my parents, decided to attend North Carolina State University. At the age of 17, I was clueless when I arrived to the College of Agriculture and Life Sciences, and eventually decided to major in Biochemistry.

In 2001, I graduated from North Carolina State University with a Bachelor's of Science in (Structural and Molecular) Biochemistry, and gained interest in understanding the human body, its reactions to different stimuli and figuring out solutions to major diseases through a biochemical viewpoint. I worked at aaiPharma Inc. after my graduation in a phase I clinic as a laboratory technician and administrative assistant, and was introduced to a great doctor, research nurse and staff who believed that I could become something more than a laboratory processor.

I then applied to medical schools in Europe and found myself in the University of Zagreb Faculty of Medicine, which was previously partnered with Harvard Medical International. As I started my medical education and explored possibilities in medicine, I became interested in internal medicine, emergency medicine, pathology, general practice, alternative medicine, and public health.

I went back to Malaysia after getting my degree as a Doctor of Medicine from the University of Zagreb Faculty of Medicine, and was trying to find employment opportunities in clinical research or medical journalism, something I became interested in when I was in medical school. I could not find a job as my degree was not recognized by the Malaysian Medical Council. In the meantime, I built aspirations to work in or start an NGO or a NPO, so that my life would have that underlying purpose.

After moving back to Zagreb and changing Croatia's laws with a colleague, I completed my internship position at KBC Sestre Milosrdnice and passed the state licensing examination in April 2013. I accepted a position in Zadar, Croatia as a Doctor of Medicine in Emergency Medicine for Zadarska Županija, then moved to Martinščica on Cres Island to work as a Primary Care Physician. Since then, I worked in emergency departments and clinics in various rural and border areas in Croatia, giving me extensive experience in rural medicine, emergency medicine, trauma response and primary care in hard-to-reach places.

Read more at yeopazman.wordpress.com